hamlyn

QuickCook
Recipes for Kids

Recipes by Emma Frost

Every dish, three ways – you choose!
30 minutes | 20 minutes | 10 minutes

An Hachette UK Company
www.hachette.co.uk

First published in Great Britain in 2013 by Hamlyn,
a division of Octopus Publishing Group Ltd
Endeavour House, 189 Shaftesbury Avenue
London WC2H 8JY
www.octopusbooks.co.uk

ISBN 978-0-600-62526-1

A CIP catalogue record for this book is available from the British Library

Printed and bound in China

10 9 8 7 6 5 4 3 2 1

Both metric and imperial measurements are given for the recipes. Use one set of
measures only, not a mixture of both.

Standard level spoon measurements are used in all recipes
1 tablespoon = 15 ml
1 teaspoon = 5 ml

Ovens should be preheated to the specified temperature. If using a fan-assisted oven,
follow the manufacturer's instructions for adjusting the time and temperature. Grills
should also be preheated.

This book includes dishes made with nuts and nut derivatives. It is advisable for
those with known allergic reactions to nuts and nut derivatives and those who may
be potentially vulnerable to these allergies, such as pregnant and nursing mothers,
invalids, the elderly, babies and children, to avoid dishes made with nuts and nut oils.

It is also prudent to check the labels of prepreared ingredients for the possible
inclusion of nut derivatives.

The Department of Health advises that eggs should not be consumed raw. This book
contains some dishes made with raw or lightly cooked eggs. It is prudent for more
vulnerable people such as pregnant and nursing mothers, invalids, the elderly, babies
and young children to avoid uncooked or lightly cooked dishes made with eggs.

Contents

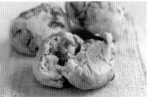
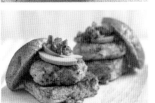
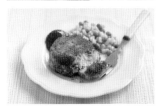
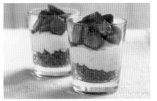
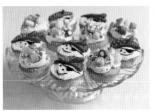

Introduction

30 20 10 – Quick, Quicker, Quickest

This book offers a new and flexible approach to meal-planning for busy cooks, letting you choose the recipe option that best fits the time you have available. Inside you will find 360 dishes that will inspire and motivate you to get cooking every day of the year. All the recipes take a maximum of 30 minutes to cook. Some take as little as 20 minutes and, amazingly, many take only 10 minutes. With a bit of preparation, you can easily try out one new recipe from this book each night and slowly you will be able to build a wide and exciting portfolio of recipes to suit your needs.

How Does it Work?

Every recipe in the QuickCook series can be cooked one of three ways – a 30-minute version, a 20-minute version or a super-quick and easy 10-minute version. At the beginning of each chapter you'll find recipes listed by time. Choose a dish based on how much time you have and turn to that page.

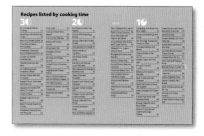

You'll find the main recipe in the middle of the page accompanied by a beautiful photograph, as well as two time-variation recipes below.

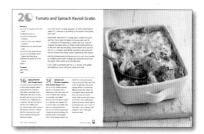

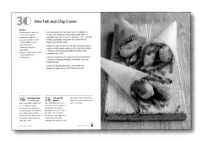

If you enjoy your chosen dish, why not go back and cook the other time-variation options at a later date? So, if you liked the 20-minute Fish and Chip Butties, but only have 10 minutes to spare this time around, you'll find a way to cook it using cheat ingredients or clever shortcuts.

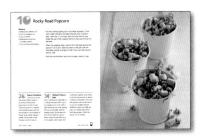

If you love the ingredients and flavours of the 10-minute Rocky Road Popcorn, why not try something more substantial like the 20-minute Popcorn Necklaces, or be inspired to make a more elaborate version, like the 30-minute Malteser and Popcorn Balls? Alternatively, browse through all 360 delicious recipes, find something that catches your eye – then cook the version that fits your time frame.

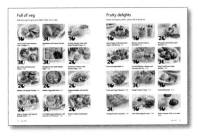

Or, for easy inspiration, turn to the gallery on pages 12–19 to get an instant overview by themes, such as Fruity delights or Classic crowd pleasers.

QuickCook online

To make life easier, you can use the special code on each recipe page to e-mail yourself a recipe card for printing, or email a text-only shopping list to your phone. Go to www.hamlynquickcook.com and enter the recipe code at the bottom of each page.

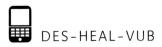

DES-HEAL-VUB

QuickCook Recipes for Kids

Cooking for our families in today's hectic times can be hard. Life is busy as we find more and more after-school activities have to be woven into our children's week. As a result, although many of us crave spending quality time together over a leisurely family meal, it often seems like there is barely enough time to eat a meal, let alone shop for it, prepare it and cook it!

Designed for busy parents in a hurry, this book includes 100 great recipes, for kids of all ages, that can be cooked in 30 minutes or less. Whether you have 30, 20 or even as few as 10 minutes available, you'll find a tasty and nutritious recipe that will suit your children's taste buds as well as fit in with your busy lives. And because children can get bored with a small repertoire, there are two variations on each recipe that can be cooked in slightly less or more time.

Can good food be fast food?

This book is simple and realistic, and the recipes are genuinely fast! It is assumed you are on your own with up to four children to cook for, and that sometimes you will have to 'cheat'. There are some ready-prepared ingredients in the recipes – shop-bought sauces, packets of flavoured grains such as rice and couscous, and purées such as garlic, lemon grass and ginger – to add instant but intense flavours to your cooking. It is also assumed that you own a few key kitchen gadgets such as an electric whisk, a small food processor and a microwave. These will save you time and enable you to experiment with many different ingredients and flavours.

Another important factor in cooking well for kids is preparation. It's tricky to find the time to sit down at the beginning of the week and plan meals for the days ahead, but it helps stress levels and the household budget if you know roughly what you are going to cook. Scanning a recipe in advance will ensure you have the necessary fresh, dried and canned ingredients to-hand.

For those moments when you discover you need to whizz up a tasty, nutritious masterpiece in minutes, always keep certain basic ingredients in the kitchen. Here are some suggestions:

- plain flour, self-raising flour and cornflour;
- dried pasta shapes, rice and couscous;
- quick protein, such as tuna, cheese, prawns and chicken;
- all types of canned beans;
- intense flavourings, such as stock cubes, soy sauce, dried herbs and spices (especially cumin, coriander, cinnamon, mixed herbs and nutmeg);
- cans of tomatoes and coconut milk;
- jars of olives, pesto and purées such as garlic and ginger;
- frozen vegetables, such as chopped spinach, peas and sweetcorn, frozen fruit such as raspberries.

It's also a good idea to buy in some vital 'cheat's' ingredients for those days when time is really stretched. Ready-rolled shortcrust and puff pastry, ready-cooked chicken, pitta breads and chapattis, custard powder, ready-prepared pizza bases and croissant dough, cooked rice and ready-made mash and cans of condensed soups are just some of the 'instant' ingredients used in the recipes.

Fast and healthy!

Being in a hurry does not mean compromising on nutritional value. Getting kids used to healthy food means they are less likely to crave bad food as they enter their teens and gives them a much better chance of growing into fit and healthy adults.

Simple changes to your buying and cooking habits will give your children the best start. One small but significant change is to cut out salt from your cooking (officially known as sodium); this is a vital mineral that helps with muscular movement, messages to the nerves, and the pH of blood. It is not necessary to add it to your cooking though. It is found naturally in every type of food and is especially high in processed foods. Salt is a taste we learn to expect; if you eradicate it from your cooking while your children are young, they quickly become used to the flavours of food without it.

Other small changes you can make include replacing canned fruits with fresh, limiting processed meats such as bacon, sausages and ham to no more than 2–3 times per week, and substituting refined white flour products such as flour, pasta and wraps with the brown/wholewheat versions.

Wholegrains will give your child slow-release energy and a host of nutrients not found in the refined versions; however, these foods have a slightly nuttier, denser flavour and take a little getting used to. Persist with the changes and your children will benefit.

Dealing with the fussy eater

The frustration felt by a parent of a fussy eater is immense; you want so much to feed your children wholesome, tasty, attractive meals. You work hard to create breakfasts, lunches, snacks and dinners that all the children will eat and enjoy, but preparing a meal that is instantly rejected is very disheartening.

You can tackle the fussy eater in a number of ways. Firstly, make them hungry! A fussy eater who is known for rejecting vegetables, and who has been snacking on sweets or crisps since they got home from school, is unlikely to dive into a bowl of veggie chilli at 6 pm with enthusiasm. Fussy eaters need snacks, but ensure they are healthy and are eaten with at least 2 hours to spare before the next meal. If your child is hungry before dinner is ready, put out a bowl of hummus and vegetable sticks. A genuinely hungry child will eat.

Secondly, get the fussy eater involved with their meal. From a young age, most kids love to cook, but we forget this as they grow up. Time pressures mean we often keep the kitchen door shut when preparing meals to save ourselves from interruptions. Remember, your children can be of help to you! If they want to get involved and time is not on your side, give them some easy jobs such as sieving the flour or cutting out the pastry circles for the mini quiches (page 66). Alternatively, get them dipping chicken strips into couscous (page 56) or cracking eggs into a bowl. If they feel involved, they are less likely to reject the end result.

Thirdly, rather than dish up a prepared meal on individual plates, let the children help themselves from a large serving bowl of food in the middle of the table. A fussy eater likes to think they have chosen their own meal – give them choice, within reason, and allow them to feel in control.

Finally, many children today are unaware of where their food comes from. Put food into its context by visiting farms and food-producers and making your children aware of what goes into making the food they are eating. If you can get into the countryside, let your kids pick their own fruit, so they know what is in season and when. Or if you can't make it to a farm, then buy peas in their shells and shell them together at the table. If you have a small patch of ground in the garden, or even a windowsill, a fun thing to do is to grow some produce at home. Courgettes, potatoes, carrots, tomatoes and certain herbs are all easy to grow. Kids love the outdoors; if they equate fruit and vegetables with the outdoor activities of sowing, growing and picking, they are much more likely to enjoy eating them.

Patience in a hurry

Fussy children, stressed parents and a lack of time are rarely a happy combination, but this book offers you over 300 delicious, quick and easy recipes that will fit your family's tastes, timings and budget. Set aside a few minutes today to choose the meals that you think will work for your kids, order your shopping online, and then among the chaos of school pick-ups and drop-offs, football training and music recitals, you will at least know that the food for next week is sorted!

Full of veg

Delicious ways to give your children their five-a-day!

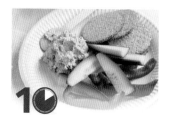
Carrot and Cumin Hummus with Crudités 42

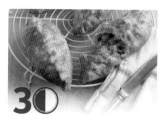
Vegetable and Cheese Pasties 70

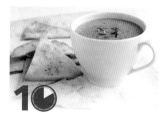
Creamy Tomato Soup with Baked Tortilla Crisps 96

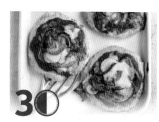
Easy Ham and Veg Scone Pizzas 100

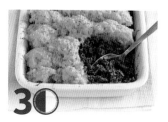
Shepherd's Pie (with Hidden Veg!) 104

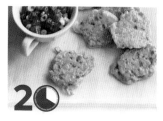
Sweetcorn Fritters with Tomato Salsa 108

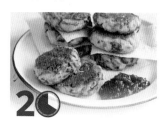
Bubble and Squeak Patties 116

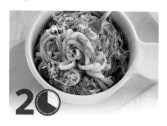
Hidden Vegetable Pasta 120

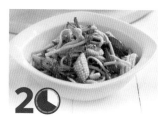
Veggie Noodles with Hoi Sin 126

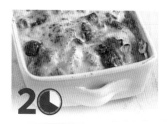
Cherry Tomato and Spinach Ravioli Gratin 130

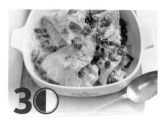
Scrambled Egg Enchiladas with Spinach and Tomatoes 164

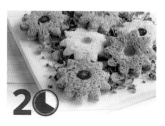
Flower Garden Sandwiches 272

Fruity delights

Sweet and savoury dishes, packed full of goodness.

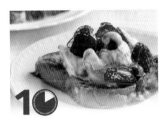

10 Spiced Eggy Fruit Bread with Yogurt and Berries 24

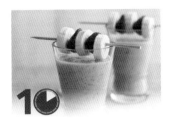

10 Banana and Strawberry Smoothie 38

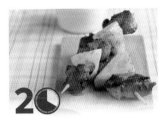

20 Pineapple and Chunky Ham Skewers 64

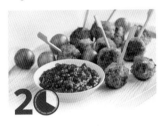

20 Pork and Apple Balls 84

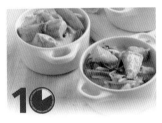

10 Curried Chicken, Mango and Coconut Stir-Fry 142

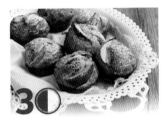

30 Peach and Brown Sugar Muffins 198

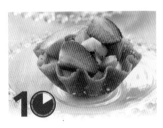

10 Fruit and Yogurt Baskets 206

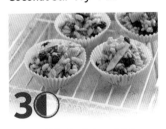

30 Mango Krispie Cakes 212

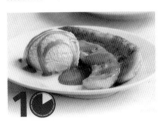

10 Caramel Bananas 214

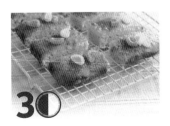

30 Orange Drizzle Tray Bake 226

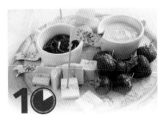

10 Chocolate Dipped Fruits 230

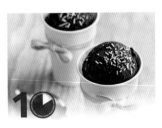

10 Quick Summer Fruit Ice Cream 238

Classic crowd pleasers

Comfort food and familar favourites to make for the masses.

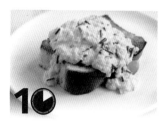

Creamy Scrambled Egg with Chives 26

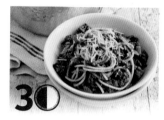

Spaghetti Bolognaise 134

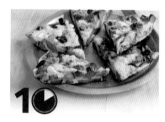

Frankfurter and Courgette Frittata 136

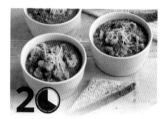

Hearty Bean, Bacon and Pasta Soup 148

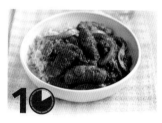

Sausage, Tomato and Pepper Pan-Fry 190

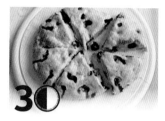

Blueberry Scones 200

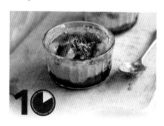

Rice Pudding and Jam Brûlée 216

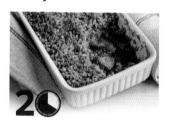

Rhubarb and Strawberry Oat Crumble 218

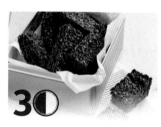

Chocolate Flapjacks 236

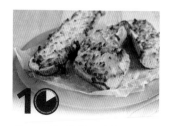

Cheesy Garlic Bread 266

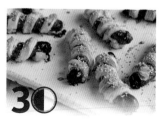

Whirly Sausage Rolls 268

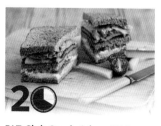

BLT Club Sandwiches 274

Give it a try

Some clever snacks, meals and puddings for tempting those taste-buds.

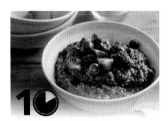

Chocolate Porridge with Berries 30

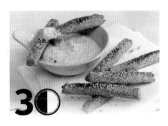

Wholemeal Cheese Straws with Pesto Dip 52

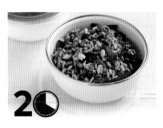

Brown Rice Salad with Peanuts and Raisins 58

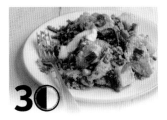

Curried Chicken Couscous Salad 68

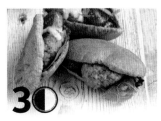

Mini Falafel Burgers 74

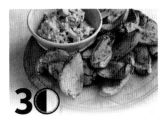

Potato Skins with Guacamole 128

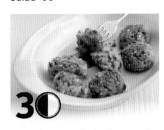

Spiced Rice and Chickpea Balls with Sweet Chilli Sauce 156

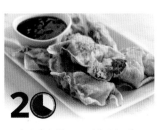

Pork Dumplings with Dipping Sauce 178

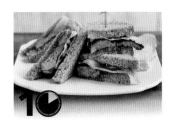

Curried Lamb Steak Sandwiches 184

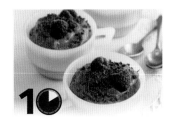

Chocolate Pots with Hidden Prunes 204

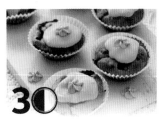

Iced Banana and Honey Buns 232

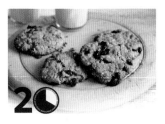

Spiced Raisin and Cranberry Cookies 240

Chicken favourites

Protein-packed and full of flavour, great chicken dishes for everyday eating.

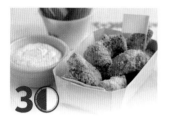

Crunchy Chicken Pesto
Dippers 56

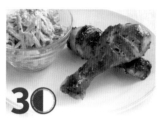

Sticky Chicken Drumsticks
with Homemade Coleslaw 72

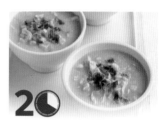

Chicken and Sweetcorn Soup
86

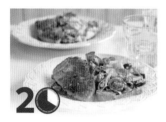

Parmesan Chicken Salad 94

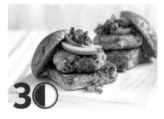

Mexican Chicken and Avocado
Burgers with Salsa 98

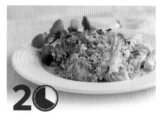

Creamy Chicken and Broccoli
Pasta Gratin 102

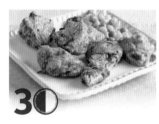

Chicken Nuggets with Sunblush
Tomato Sauce 122

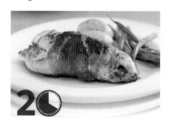

Chicken, Pesto and Bacon
Pan-Fry 132

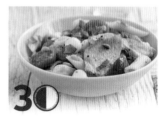

Warm Mozzarella, Chicken,
Tomato and Basil Pasta 152

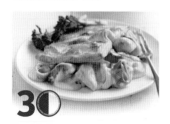

Chicken, Bacon and Leek Pies
174

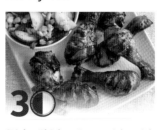

Sticky Chicken Drumsticks with
Cucumber and Sweetcorn 182

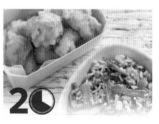

Crispy Chicken with Egg Fried
Rice 188

Fish favourites

Fried, in a pie, stir-fried or served in a cone, these are great for fish fans.

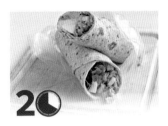

Tuna and Sweetcorn Wraps 50

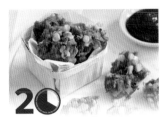

Tuna and Sweetcorn Nuggets 90

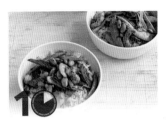

Sweet Chilli Prawn and Green Vegetable Stir-Fry 92

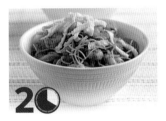

Singapore Noodles 110

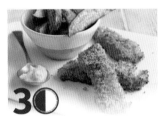

Fish Fingers with Sweet Potato Chips 112

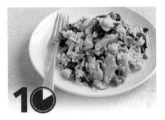

Kedgeree-Style Rice with Spinach 150

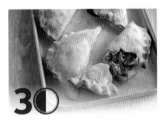

Tuna, Pepper and Cheese Calzone 162

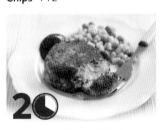

Salmon and Broccoli Fishcakes 168

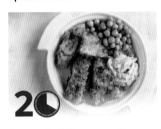

Lemon Cod Goujons with 'Caperless' Tartare Sauce 172

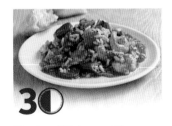

Chorizo, Chicken and Prawn Jambalaya 176

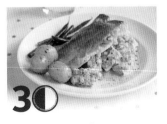

Creamy Pesto Fish Pie 180

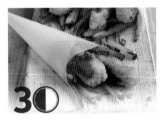

Mini Fish and Chip Cones 276

Food fun

Finger food and tasty treats to brighten up any table. Girls and boys will love these!

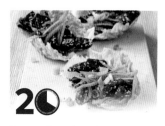

2 Honeyed Duck Strips in Lettuce 'Boats' 62

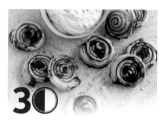

3 Marmite Pinwheels with Soft Cheese Dip 76

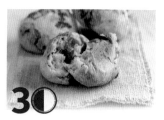

3 Pepperoni and Pepper Rolls 78

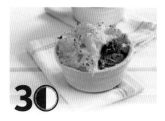

3 Creamy Pork and Apple Pies 154

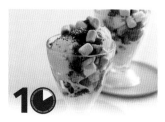

1 Strawberry Ice Cream Sundae 210

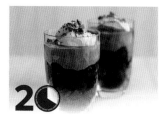

2 Chocolate Muffin and Custard Trifles 244

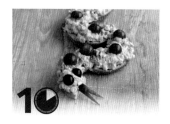

1 Slippery Snake 250

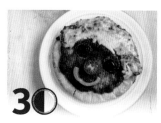

3 Pizza Bear Faces 252

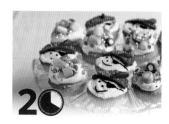

2 Pirate and Princess Cakes 256

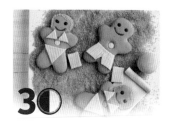

3 Gingerbread People Beach Party 258

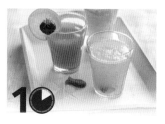

1 Mocktails 260

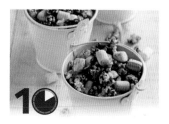

1 Rocky Road Popcorn 270

Weekend treats

Delicious food for cooking and enjoying together as a family.

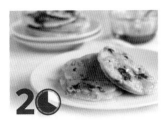

Raspberry and Oatmeal Scotch Pancakes with Syrup 36

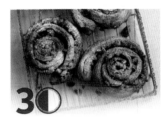

Cinnamon Buns 46

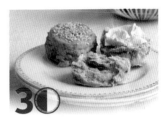

Ricotta and Tomato Scones 60

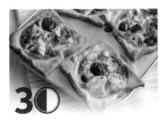

Mini Brie and Tomato Quiches 66

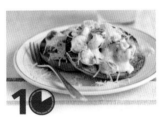

Creamy Garlic Mushroom Bagels 118

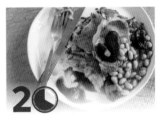

Rosti with Bacon and Mushrooms 146

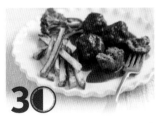

Beef Meatballs with Gravy and Baked Fries 166

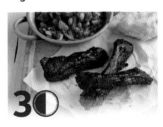

Sticky Pork Ribs with Homemade Baked Beans 186

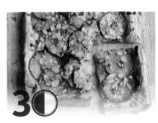

Apple and Almond Tart 222

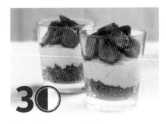

Strawberry and Lime Cheesecakes 224

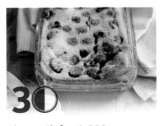

Cherry Clafouti 228

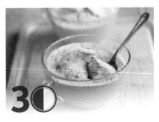

Saucy Lemon Puddings 234

QuickCook
Breakfast
& Lunchbox

Recipes listed by cooking time

30

20

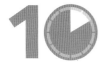

Spiced Eggy Fruit Bread with Berry Yogurt

Serves 4

2 eggs
25 g (1 oz) caster sugar
½ teaspoon ground cinnamon
4 tablespoons milk
25 g (1 oz) butter
4 slices of fruit bread
100 g (3½ oz) mixed berries
8 tablespoons thick Greek yogurt
  or fromage frais
4 teaspoons clear honey, to serve

- Beat the eggs in a bowl with the sugar, cinnamon and milk. Heat the butter in a large heavy-based frying pan. Dip the fruit bread slices, 2 at a time, into the egg mixture, covering both sides, then lift into the hot pan and fry for 1–2 minutes on each side until golden. Repeat with the remaining fruit bread slices.

- Mix half the berries into the yogurt or fromage frais.

- Serve the warm fruit bread slices with spoonfuls of the fruit yogurt, scattered with the remaining berries and drizzled with the honey.

---

2 Fruit Bread and Berry Pan Pudding

Tear 4 slices of fruit bread into bite-sized pieces. Put 2 eggs, 25 g (1 oz) caster sugar, ½ teaspoon ground cinnamon and 150 ml (¼ pint) milk into a bowl and mix well. Add the bread to the bowl and set aside to soak up the milk for 5 minutes. Heat 25 g (1 oz) butter in a medium heavy-based frying pan and pour in the bread and milk mixture. Scatter over 50 g (2 oz) mixed berries. Cook over a medium heat for 3–4 minutes until the base is set. Place the pan under a preheated medium grill (keeping the handle away from the heat) and cook for 4–5 minutes until the top is set. Serve warm spooned into serving bowls with yogurt for a warming breakfast or dessert.

3 Berry Bread and Butter Puddings

Spread 6 slices of fruit bread with 25 g (1 oz) butter, then cut them into triangles. Place half the bread in the base of a lightly buttered ovenproof gratin dish, then scatter over 50 g (2 oz) berries. Put the remaining bread slices over the top. Mix 2 eggs with 150 ml (¼ pint) milk, ½ teaspoon ground cinnamon and 25 g (1 oz) caster sugar in a jus, then pour over the bread slices and fruit. Bake in a preheated oven, 180°C (350°F), Gas Mark 4, for 15–20 minutes until golden and just setting. Serve spooned into serving bowls with honey and yogurt, if liked.

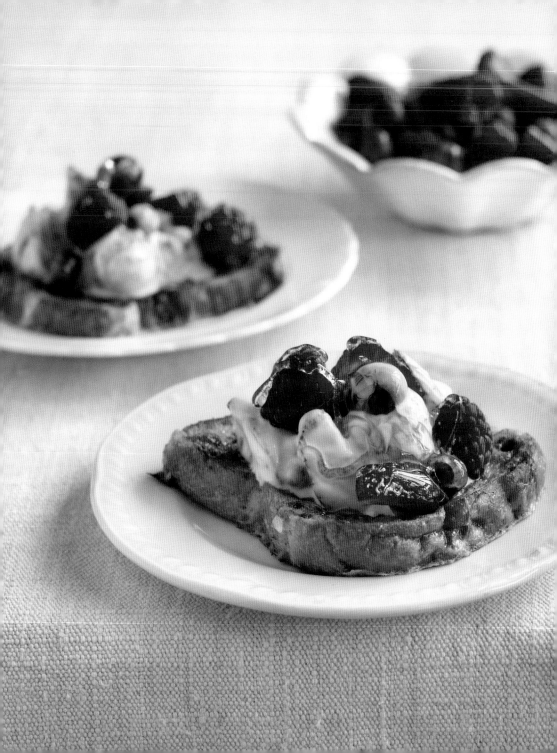

10 Creamy Scrambled Egg with Chives

Serves 2

2 thick slices of brioche
4 eggs
6 tablespoons water
15 g (½ oz) butter
2 tablespoons finely grated
   Parmesan cheese
4 tablespoons crème fraîche
2 tablespoons snipped chives
pepper

- Lightly toast the brioche slices under a preheated grill until just golden, then turn over and lightly toast on the other side. Keep warm.

- Break the eggs into a saucepan, add the measurement water and butter and beat together. Season generously with pepper.

- Cook over a medium heat, stirring continuously, until just beginning to scramble. Add the Parmesan and continue to cook, stirring and watching carefully, taking care not to overcook the eggs, until the eggs are soft and slightly runny. Remove from the heat when almost cooked and stir in the crème fraîche and chives.

- Pile on to the warm brioche slices and serve warm with a sauce of your choice, if liked.

20 Chive and Parmesan Eggy

Brioche Mix 3 eggs in a bowl with 150 ml (¼ pint) milk, 2 tablespoons Parmesan cheese and 4 tablespoons chopped chives. Add 4 slices of brioche and leave to soak up the egg mixture for 3–4 minutes. Heat 2 tablespoons olive oil in a large heavy-based frying pan. Using a fish slice, lift 2 of the brioche slices from the egg mixture and cook over a high heat for 2 minutes on each side until golden. Repeat with the other 2 slices. Serve 2 per person scattered with a little more Parmesan and chopped chives, if liked.

30 Baked Eggs with Spinach and Chives

Lightly grease 2 ramekins with 15 g (½ oz) butter, add 1 tablespoon finely grated Parmesan cheese to each and knock around the ramekin to coat. Place 150 g (5 oz) washed spinach leaves in a saucepan over a high heat and stir for 2–3 minutes until wilted. Remove from the heat, put the spinach in a sieve and squeeze out any excess water. Divide between the ramekins. Break 1 egg into each of the ramekins, then top each with a pinch of grated nutmeg and ½ tablespoon chopped chives on each.

Bake in a preheated oven, 180°C (350°F), Gas Mark 4, for 15–20 minutes until the eggs are just set. Serve with brioche slices or crusty bread.

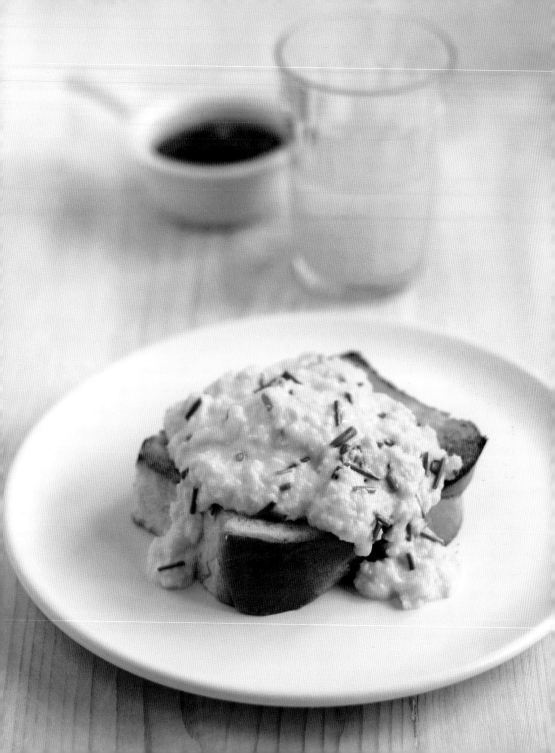

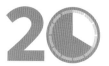

Sausage, Bacon and Tomato Frittata

Serves 4

flour, for dusting
175 g (6 oz) sausagemeat
2 tablespoons olive oil
6 streaky bacon rashers, snipped into pieces
4 vine tomatoes, cut into wedges
6 eggs
pepper
4 tablespoons chopped parsley
slices of toast, to serve

- Using lightly floured hands, divide the sausagemeat into 8 pieces. Shape into very rough balls, then lightly flatten.

- Heat the oil in a heavy-based nonstick frying pan. Add the sausagemeat patties and cook over a medium heat for 5 minutes, turning once, until golden and cooked through. Add the bacon and cook for a further 3 minutes until cooked.

- Add the tomatoes, remove from the heat and evenly spread the ingredients around the pan.

- Beat the eggs with the parsley, then season with pepper and pour into the pan. Return to the heat and cook over a medium heat for 3–4 minutes until the base is set. Place the pan under a preheated hot grill (keeping the handle away from the heat) and cook for 3–4 minutes until it is set.

- Divide into wedges and serve with slices of toast.

 Pan-Fried Egg, Sausage and Tomato on Toast Heat 2 tablespoons olive oil in a frying pan. Using lightly floured hands, divide 175 g (6 oz) sausagemeat into 8 small balls; press into patties. Cook the patties in a little oil over a medium heat for 4–5 minutes, turning once, until cooked, adding 4 halved vine tomatoes for the final 2 minutes. In a separate nonstick frying pan heat 1 tablespoon olive oil and fry 2 eggs over medium heat for 2–3 minutes. Serve all on toast.

 Bacon and Tomato Quiche Unroll 1 ready-rolled shortcrust pastry sheet and use to line a 30 x 20 cm (12 x 8 inch) shallow tin. Scatter 100 g (4 oz) precooked bacon, broken into small pieces, and 5 vine tomatoes, cut into wedges, into the tin. Beat 6 eggs with 3 tablespoons chopped parsley and plenty of pepper in a jug, then pour over the bacon and tomato. Bake in a preheated oven, 200°C (400°F), Gas Mark 6, for 20 minutes until well risen and golden. The quiche will sink as you remove it from the oven. Serve cut into wedges. A great breakfast to eat on the move!

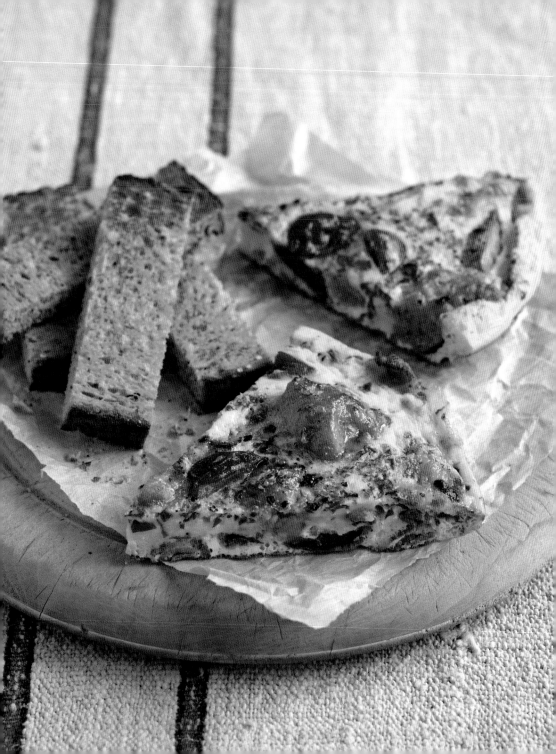

10 Chocolate Porridge with Berries

Serves 2

600 ml (1 pint) milk (or rice milk
 for a dairy-free option)
100 g (3½ oz) porridge oats
3 tablespoons cocoa powder, plus
 extra for dusting (optional)
4 tablespoons soft brown sugar
75 g (3 oz) mixed berries
2 tablespoons maple syrup

· Place the milk in a heavy-based saucepan with the oats
 and bring to the boil. Add the cocoa powder and sugar,
 then reduce the heat and simmer for 6–7 minutes, stirring
 occasionally, until the oats have swollen and the porridge
 has thickened, adding a little water to loosen if necessary.

· Mix the berries with the maple syrup. Serve the porridge
 in warmed serving bowls with the berries spooned into
 the centre. Dust with cocoa powder, if liked.

20 Chocolate and Fruit Muesli

Roughly chop 50 g (2 oz) hazelnuts and lightly toast the under a preheated hot grill for 5–10 minutes of until golden brown. Place 300 g (10 oz) porridge oats in a large bowl, add 2 tablespoons cocoa powder and toss well. Roughly chop 125 g (4 oz) fresh or dried dates and add to the bowl along with the toasted hazelnuts. Roughly crumble 75 g (3 oz) banana chips and toss into the mix. Add 1 tablespoon hemp seeds and 50 g (2 oz) bran flakes and toss again. Spoon a little into a cereal bowl and pour over milk to cover. Leave to stand for 5 minutes to allow the porridge to swell, then add a little more milk to taste. Sprinkle with golden caster sugar to serve.

30 Chocolate and Raisin Porridge

Bars Place 300 ml (½ pint) boiling water in a saucepan with 100 g (3½ oz) porridge oats, 50 g (2 oz) raisins, 3 tablespoons cocoa powder and 4 tablespoons soft brown sugar and bring back to the boil. Reduce the heat to a simmer and stir continuously for about 2–3 minutes until very thick. Transfer to a 20 cm (8 inch) square cake tin and smooth the top. Chill for 20 minutes until solid, then cut into 12 squares or bars to serve (these will keep for up to 3 days refrigerated in an airtight container).

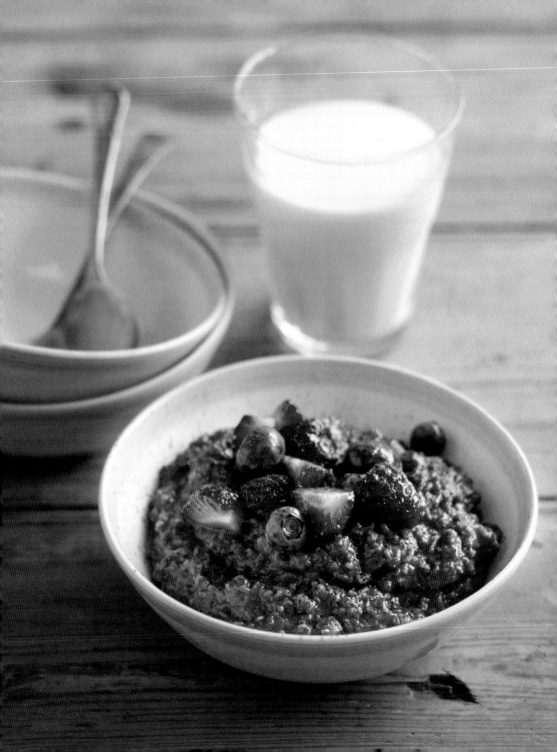

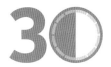

Wholemeal Cheese and Bacon Breakfast Muffins

Makes 12

375 g (12 oz) wholemeal
self-raising flour
1 teaspoon baking powder
1 teaspoon bicarbonate of soda
2 teaspoons mustard powder
125 g (4 oz) Cheddar cheese,
grated
50 g (2 oz) cooked bacon
pieces, chopped
2 eggs
75 ml (3 fl oz) vegetable oil
200 ml (7 fl oz) milk
salt and pepper

- Line a 12-hole muffin tin with 12 paper muffin cases.

- Sift the flour, baking powder, bicarbonate of soda and mustard powder into a bowl and season with a pinch of salt and pepper. Stir in the cheese and bacon pieces.

- Mix together the egg with the oil and milk in a jug, then pour into the dry ingredients and mix well, adding a little milk if the mixture is too dry.

- Divide the mixture evenly between the paper cases and bake in a preheated oven, 180°C (350°F), Gas Mark 4, for 20–25 minutes until golden and risen.

- Serve warm if possible, but they are equally delicious cold.

 Cheese and Bacon Pan Scones

Place 250 g (8 oz) wholemeal self-raising flour in a bowl with a pinch of salt, 25 g (1 oz) grated Cheddar cheese, 25 g (1 oz) finely broken cooked bacon pieces, 1 egg and 275 ml (9 fl oz) milk and mix well. Brush a frying pan with a little melted butter. Drop small rounds of the mixture from a spoon or small ladle into the pan and cook over a medium heat for 2 minutes, then turn the scones over with a palette knife and cook for a further 1–2 minutes until golden. Repeat with the remaining mixture to make 8 scones. Serve warm.

 Cheese and Bacon Tray Bake

Place 250 g (8 oz) self-raising wholemeal flour in a bowl with 1 teaspoon baking powder and 1 teaspoon mustard powder. Mix in 75 g (3 oz) grated Cheddar cheese and 50 g (2 oz) chopped cooked bacon pieces and stir well. Beat 1 egg with 50 ml (2 fl oz) vegetable oil and 50 ml (2 fl oz) milk in a jug, then pour into the dry ingredients and mix well. Pour into a well-greased 18 x 28 cm (7 x 11 inch) Swiss roll tin and bake in a preheated oven, 180°C (350°F), Gas Mark 4, for 12–15 minutes until well risen and golden.

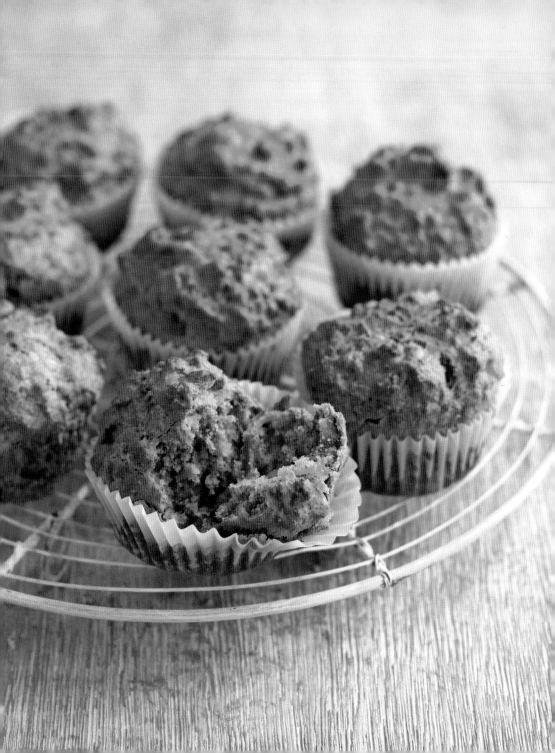

30 On-the-Go Granola Breakfast Bars

Makes 9

75 g (3 oz) butter, plus extra for greasing

75 ml (3 fl oz) clear honey

½ teaspoon ground cinnamon

100 g (3½ oz) ready-to-eat dried apricots, roughly chopped

50 g (2 oz) ready-to-eat dried papaya or mango, roughly chopped

50 g (2 oz) raisins

4 tablespoons mixed seeds, such as pumpkin, sesame, sunflower

50 g (2 oz) pecan nuts, roughly broken

150 g (5 oz) porridge oats

- Grease a shallow 20 cm (8 inch) square tin.

- Place the butter and honey in a saucepan and bring to the boil, stirring continuously, until the mixture bubbles. Add the cinnamon, dried fruit, seeds and nuts, then stir and heat for 1 minute. Remove from the heat and add the oats. Stir well, then transfer to the prepared tin and press down well. Bake in a preheated oven, 190°C (375°F), Gas Mark 5, for 15 minutes until the top is just beginning to brown.

- Leave to cool in the tin, then cut into 9 squares or bars to serve.

1 Granola, Yogurt and Fruit Layer

Divide 200 g (7 oz) ready-made granola cereal between 4 glasses and top each with 4 tablespoons Greek yogurt. Chop 75 g (3 oz) mixed ready-to-eat dried fruits, such as mango, apricots and raisins, and toss with 2 pinches of ground cinnamon. Spoon on top of the yogurt and drizzle each with 1 teaspoon clear honey to serve.

2 Homemade Granola Cereal

Place 275 g (9 oz) porridge oats in a bowl with 2 tablespoons vegetable oil, 6 tablespoons clear honey, ½ teaspoon ground cinnamon and 1 teaspoon vanilla extract and stir well to coat. Spread on to a baking sheet and bake in a preheated oven, 180°C (350°F), Gas Mark 4, for 10–15 minutes until lightly golden. Stir in 75 g (3 oz) chopped ready-to-eat dried apricots, 75 g (3 oz) ready-to-eat dried papaya or mango, 75 g (3 oz) raisins and 3 tablespoons mixed seeds. Serve in bowls with milk.

KID-BREA-LUE

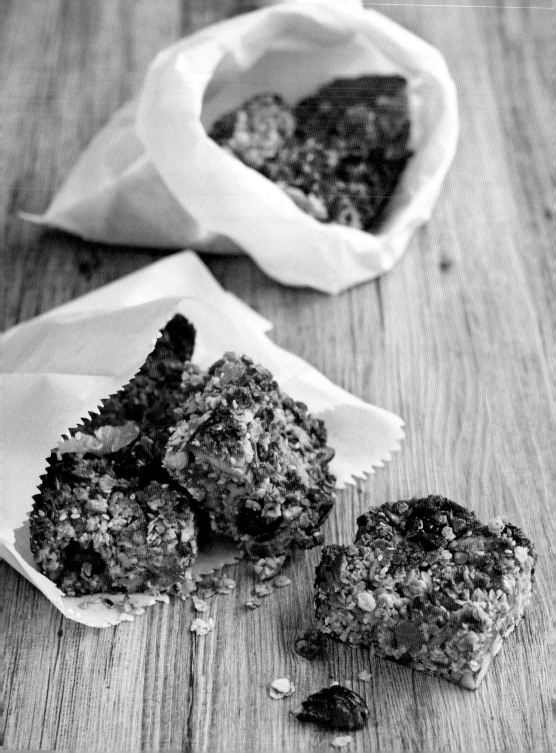

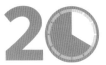

Raspberry and Oatmeal Scotch Pancakes

Makes 8

125 g (4 oz) self-raising flour
2 tablespoons golden caster sugar
2 tablespoons oatmeal
1 egg, beaten
½ teaspoon vanilla extract
150 ml (¼ pint) milk
75 g (3 oz) raspberries, halved
oil, for frying
8 tablespoons maple syrup, to serve

- Place the flour in a bowl with the sugar and oatmeal and stir well. Make a well in the centre and set aside. Beat together the egg, vanilla extract and milk in a jug, then pour into the dry ingredients and beat lightly to make a batter the consistency of thick cream. Carefully fold in the raspberries.

- Lightly oil a heavy-based frying pan or flat griddle pan. Drop tablespoons of the batter on to the pan surface until covered, and cook over a medium heat for 1–2 minutes until bubbles rise to the surface and burst. Turn the pancakes over and cook for a further 1–2 minutes until golden and set. Remove from the pan and keep warm. Repeat with the remaining batter to make 8 pancakes.

- Serve warm, on warmed plates, with 1 tablespoon maple syrup spooned over each.

Raspberry Pancake Towers

Lightly toast 8 plain scotch pancakes or raisin and lemon pancakes under a preheated hot grill for 1–2 minutes on each side until warm and pale golden. Place 1 on a warmed serving plate and top with 1 tablespoon raspberry conserve and 4–5 raspberries. Top with another warm pancake, a dollop of natural yogurt and a drizzle of maple syrup. Repeat with the remaining pancakes.

Raspberry and Oatmeal Bake

Put 175 g (6 oz) self-raising flour into a bowl with 3 tablespoons golden caster sugar and 3 tablespoons oatmeal. Beat 2 eggs with ½ teaspoon vanilla extract and 200 ml (7 fl oz) milk, then add to the dry ingredients and beat well. Pour into a well-greased shallow ovenproof dish and scatter over 150 g (5 oz) raspberries. Mix 2 tablespoons golden caster sugar with ½ teaspoon ground cinnamon and scatter over the top. Bake in a preheated oven, 200°C (400°F), Gas Mark 6, for 20 minutes until well risen and golden. Serve warm as a delicious breakfast with spoonfuls of Greek yogurt, if liked.

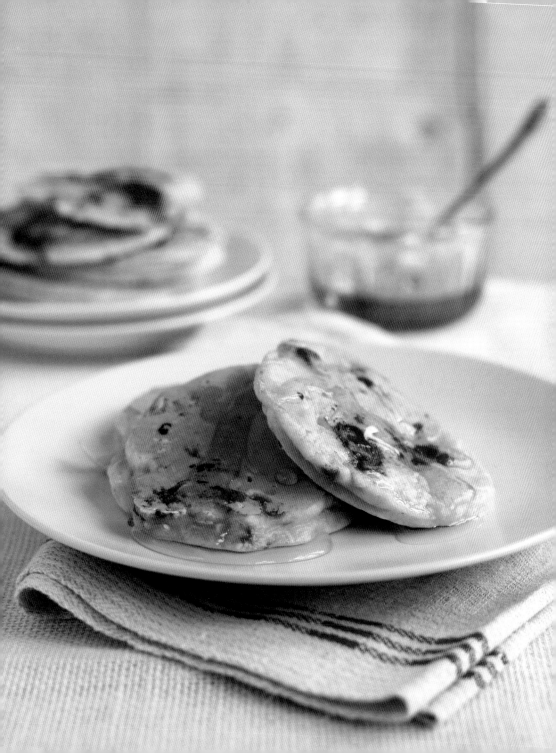

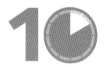 # Banana and Strawberry Smoothie

Serves 4

2 ripe bananas, roughly chopped
175 g (6 oz) strawberries, hulled
300 ml (½ pint) water
4 tablespoons fromage frais
2 tablespoons maple syrup

To serve

banana slices
strawberry halves

- Place the bananas in a food processor with the strawberries and milk. Whizz until almost smooth. Add the fromage frais and maple syrup and whizz for a short blast to mix.

- Pour into 4 small glasses and decorate each with a cocktail stick threaded with banana slices and strawberry halves for the children to dip.

 Warm Banana and Strawberry Breakfast Fools Heat 15 g (½ oz) butter in a large heavy-based frying pan and cook 2 roughly chopped bananas for 4 minutes until warm and golden. Add 6 strawberries, hulled and roughly chopped, and cook for 1 minute. Add 2 tablespoons maple syrup and toss, then cook for a further 1 minute. Serve spooned into 4 bowls, each topped with 4 tablespoons fromage frais. Scatter with a little muesli, if liked.

 Ice-Cold Banana and Strawberry Shakes Put 2 bananas into a food processor with 300 ml (½ pint) milk and 175 g (6 oz) hulled strawberries and blend until smooth. Add 12 ice cubes and whizz again until the ice is crushed finely within the shake. Pour into a shallow container and freeze for 15 minutes until thicker. Pour into glasses and decorate with cocktail sticks threaded with colourful fruit pieces of your choice.

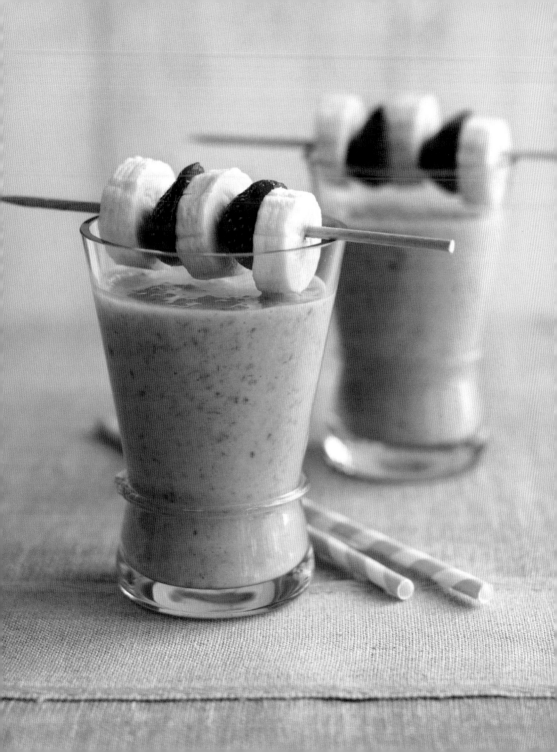

30 Savoury Cheese and Ham Croissants

Makes 6

butter, for greasing
250 g (8 oz) can croissant dough
12 slices of wafer-thin ham
6 thin slices of Gruyère or
    Emmenthal cheese
1 tablespoon Dijon mustard
beaten egg, to glaze
1 tablespoon grated Parmesan
    cheese

- Lightly grease 2 baking sheets.

- Tear the croissant dough along the perforations. For each croissant, unroll and lay 2 slices of ham on top of the dough, trying to keep the ham within the dough's outline, then lay 1 cheese slice over the top (this needs to be thin to be able to roll). Lightly spread with the mustard.

- Roll up the croissants, gently curl into a crescent shape and place on the baking sheets. Brush with beaten egg, then sprinkle with the Parmesan.

- Bake in a preheated oven, 200°C (400°F), Gas Mark 6, for 10–15 minutes until well risen and golden. Serve warm.

 Quick Cheese and Ham Croissants

Cut 4 ready-made croissants in half horizontally. Fill each with 2 slices of wafer-thin ham, 1 thin slice of Gruyère or Emmenthal cheese and 2 thick tomato slices. Place on a baking sheet and bake in a preheated oven, 200°C (400°F), Gas Mark 6, for 5 minutes until warm, then serve.

 Cheesy Croissant Pinwheels

Place a 250 g (8 oz) can croissant dough on a chopping board. Using a sharp knife, cut the dough into 15 x 1 cm (½ inch) thick pinwheels and place on a lightly greased baking sheet, cut side up. Brush each with a little beaten egg, then scatter with 3 tablespoons grated Parmesan cheese. Bake in a preheated oven, 200°C (400°F), Gas Mark 6, for 10–15 minutes until golden and lightly puffed. Serve warm with tomato ketchup for dipping.

KID-BREA-VYA

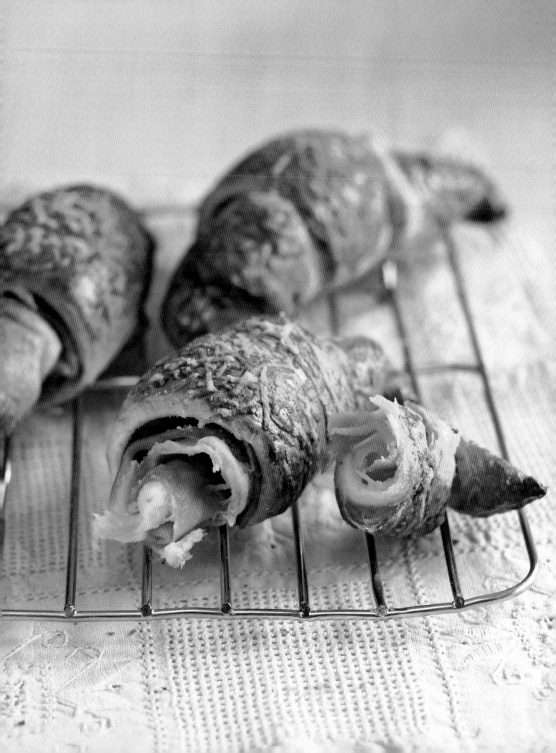

Carrot and Cumin Hummus with Crudités

Serves 4

250 g (8 oz) carrots, peeled and roughly chopped into bite-sized pieces

1 tablespoon cumin seeds

3 tablespoons olive oil

400 g (13 oz) can chickpeas, drained

4 tablespoons tahini paste

1 teaspoon ground coriander

salt and pepper

To serve

oatcakes (optional)

cucumber sticks

red pepper slices

- Put the carrots into a frying pan with the cumin seeds and oil and cook over a high heat for 5 minutes until the carrots have turned golden in places, without burning the seeds.

- Remove from the heat and place in a food processor with the chickpeas, tahini paste and coriander. Season well with salt and pepper and whizz until smooth, adding a little cold water to loosen if necessary. Transfer to a serving bowl.

- Serve with red pepper slices and cucumber sticks, and oatcakes, if liked.

 Roasted Cumin Carrots and Chickpeas Place 375 g (12 oz) peeled and roughly chopped carrots in a baking tin with 4 tablespoons olive oil and 1 tablespoon cumin seeds and toss to coat the carrots in the seeds. Add a 400 g (13 oz) can chickpeas, rinsed and drained, scatter over 2 tablespoons sesame seeds and roast at the top of a preheated oven, 200°C (400°F), Gas Mark 6, for 15 minutes until hot. Serve with crusty bread.

Roasted Carrot, Cumin and Feta Couscous Place 375 g (12 oz) peeled and chopped carrots in a baking tin with 4 tablespoons olive oil and 1 tablespoon cumin seeds and toss well. Roast in a preheated oven, 200°C (400°F), Gas Mark 6, for 15 minutes until the carrots are pale golden in places. Put 125 g (4 oz) couscous in a mixing bowl, cover with hot water and set aside for 15 minutes to swell. Meanwhile, crumble 200 g (7 oz) feta cheese into a serving bowl, add ¼ roughly chopped cucumber and mix with 1 teaspoon ground coriander. Add the swollen couscous and roasted carrots, toss together and serve.

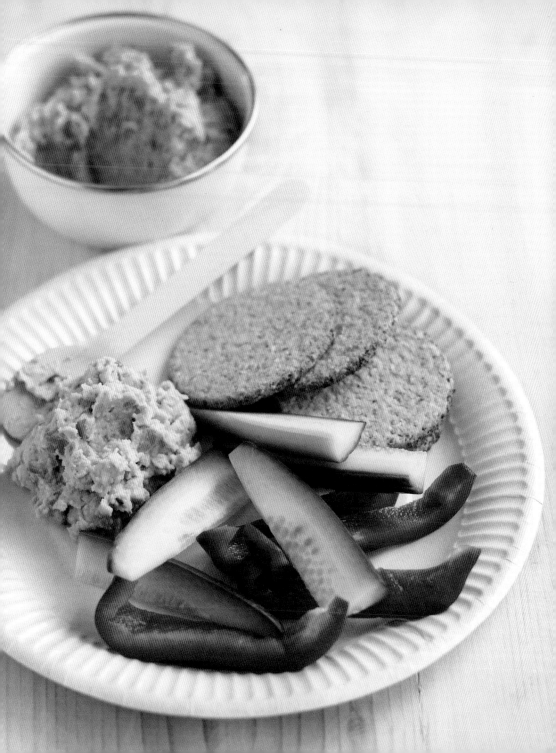

30 Sausage and Tomato Puff Pastry Turnover

Makes 4

375 g (12 oz) ready-rolled puff
    pastry
250 g (8 oz) sausagemeat
1 tablespoon wholegrain mustard
1 tablespoon chopped parsley
flour, for dusting
4 slices of tomato
beaten egg, to glaze
baked beans, to serve (optional)

- Unroll the pastry and cut into 4 equal rectangles. Place the sausagemeat in a bowl with the mustard and parsley and mix well. Using lightly floured hands, divide the sausagemeat into 4 pieces, then shape each into a rough square.

- Place 1 square at an angle in the centre of 1 pastry rectangle, then place a tomato slice on top. Fold the corners of the pastry up and over the sausagemeat to form an envelope shape. Place on a baking sheet and brush with beaten egg. Repeat with the remaining ingredients to make 4 turnovers.

- Bake in a preheated oven, 200°C (400°F), Gas Mark 6, for 15–20 minutes until well risen and golden. Serve warm with hot baked beans, if liked.

10 Cheesy Sausage and Tomato Rolls

Place 4 ready-cooked sausage rolls on a baking sheet. Lay a slice of tomato on top of each and sprinkle each with 1 teaspoon grated Parmesan cheese. Bake in a preheated oven, 200°C (400°F), Gas Mark 6, for 8 minutes until hot. Serve with hot baked beans, if liked.

20 Sausage, Tomato and Bean Puffs

Unroll 175 g (6 oz) ready-rolled puff pastry, cut into 4 equal rectangles and place on a baking sheet. Prick all over with a fork, then brush with beaten egg. Bake in a preheated oven, 200°C (400°F), Gas Mark 6, for 10–12 minutes until golden and well puffed. Meanwhile heat 1 tablespoon oil in a frying pan and cook 4 chipolata sausages for 8–10 minutes until golden and cooked through. Add 4 tomato halves, cut side down, for the final 3–4 minutes of cooking to soften and warm. Heat a 400 g (13 oz) can baked beans in a separate saucepan for 2–3 minutes until hot, stirring occasionally. Serve the warm pastry rectangles on a plate, each piled with 1 sausage, 1 tomato half and beans.

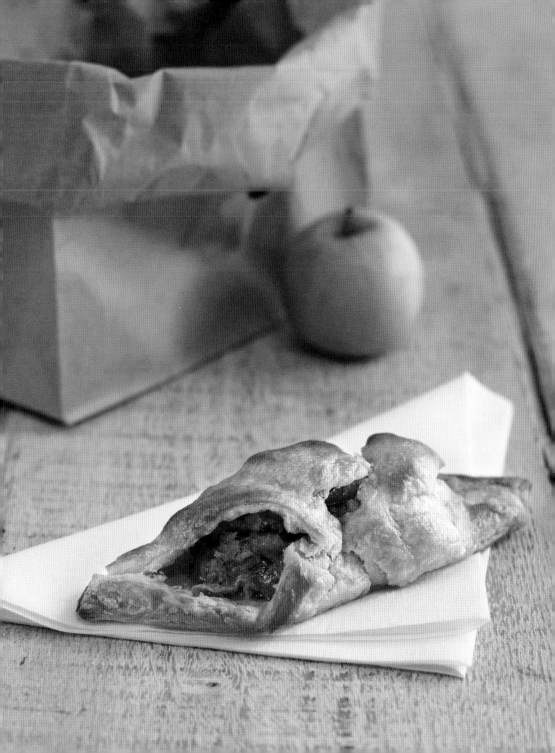

30 ⬤ Cinnamon Buns

Makes 8

4 tablespoons softened butter, plus extra for greasing

250 g (8 oz) can croissant dough

6 tablespoons soft brown sugar

3 teaspoons ground cinnamon

75 g (3 oz) pecan nuts, roughly chopped (optional)

2 tablespoons icing sugar, for dusting

- Lightly grease 2 baking sheets.

- Unroll the croissant dough on a chopping board. Place the butter, sugar and cinnamon in a bowl and beat well with a wooden spoon until soft and well blended. Spread the cinnamon butter evenly over the croissant dough, right to the edges. Sprinkle over the chopped pecans, if using, then tightly roll up the dough.

- Cut the log into 4 thick pinwheels and place well apart on the prepared baking sheets. Bake in a preheated oven, 200°C (400°F), Gas Mark 6, for 15–20 minutes until well risen and golden. Serve warm, dusted with icing sugar.

 Toasted Fruit Bread with Cinnamon Butter Cut 8 thick slices of good-quality fruit bread and cook under a preheated grill for about 2 minutes on each side until golden and lightly toasted. Meanwhile, beat 2 tablespoons butter with 2 tablespoons soft brown sugar and 1 teaspoon ground cinnamon. Spread the butter over the toasted fruit bread and serve warm with the butter melted in.

Croissant Twists with Warm Cinnamon Butter Unroll a 250 g (8 oz) can croissant dough on a chopping board. Cut into 8 strips across its width, twist each one several times and place on a nonstick baking sheet. Bake in a preheated oven, 200°C (400°F), Gas Mark 6, for 15 minutes until golden and cooked through. Meanwhile, heat 125 g (4 oz) unsalted butter in a saucepan until just beginning to melt. Transfer to a bowl and beat with 3 teaspoons ground cinnamon and 5 tablespoons soft brown sugar until warm, soft and light. Place in a serving bowl and serve with the warm twists to dip in or spread over.

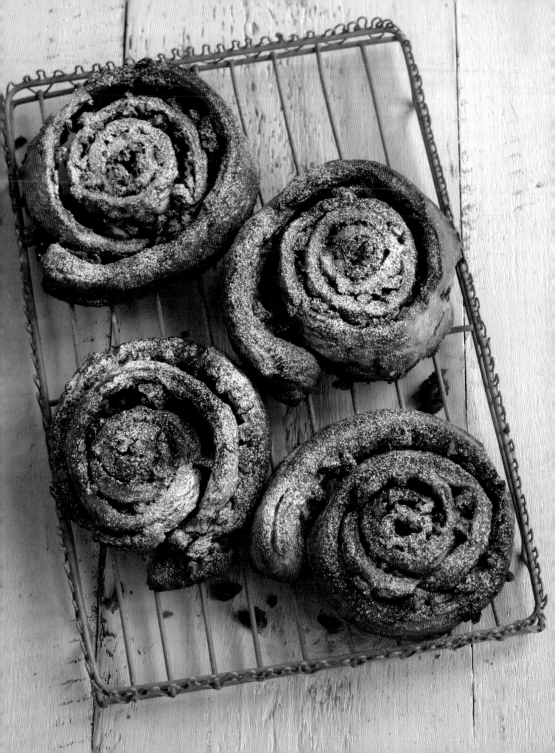

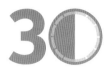 # Sausage, Sage and Onion Rolls

Makes 8

1 tablespoon olive oil
½ small red onion, finely chopped
400 g (13 oz) sausagemeat
1 tablespoon wholegrain mustard
1 tablespoon chopped sage
375 g (12 oz) ready-rolled
   shortcrust pastry
flour, for dusting
beaten egg, to glaze
apple sauce or tomato ketchup,
   to serve

- Heat the oil in a large heavy-based frying pan and cook the onion for 5 minutes over a medium heat until soft.

- Meanwhile, place the sausagemeat in a bowl with the mustard and sage and mash together well. Add the onion and mix together.

- Unroll the pastry on a floured board. Shape the sausagemeat into a long sausage shape, the length of the pastry, and place in the centre. Lightly brush one of the long edges of the pastry with beaten egg, fold the opposite edge of the pastry over the sausagemeat and press to seal. Using a fork, mark the edge to ensure the seal is made. Cut the long sausage roll into 8 equal pieces and place on a baking sheet. Score the tops, brush with beaten egg and bake in a preheated oven, 220°C (425°F), Gas Mark 7, for 15 minutes until golden and cooked. Serve with apple sauce or ketchup.

 ### Sausage, Sage and Onion Bread Rollies

Heat 1 tablespoon olive oil in a small frying pan and cook ½ small thinly sliced red onion for 5 minutes over a medium heat until softened, stirring occasionally. Meanwhile, cook 4 chipolata sausages under a preheated hot grill for 8 minutes, turning frequently, until golden and cooked through. Carefully slice the crusts off 4 slices of wholemeal bread. Spread one side of each bread slice with 1 tablespoon wholegrain mustard and 1 teaspoon tomato ketchup. Sprinkle each with a pinch of dried sage, scatter with a quarter of the onion and place 1 hot sausage on top. Roll the bread tightly around the sausages and secure with cocktail sticks (remove the sticks before serving). Serve with apple sauce or tomato ketchup to dip.

 ### Sausage, Sage and Onion Patties

Heat 1 tablespoon olive oil in a frying pan and cook 1 small finely chopped red onion for 3 minutes. Transfer to a bowl, add 500 g (1 lb) sausagemeat, 1 tablespoon wholegrain mustard and 1 tablespoon chopped sage and mash to mix. Season, then stir in 1 egg yolk and 6 tablespoons breadcrumbs. Divide into 8, shape each piece into a ball, then press to form rounded patties. Heat 2 tablespoons olive oil in a heavy-based frying pan and cook the patties over a medium heat for 10–12 minutes, turning until golden and cooked.

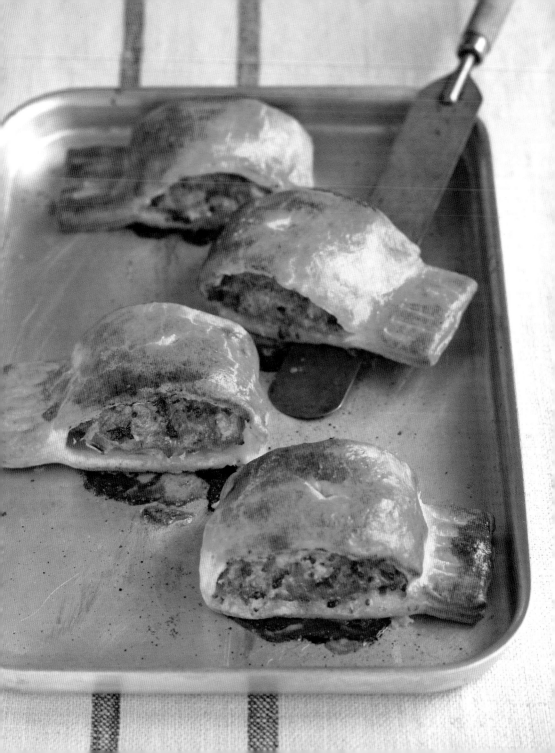

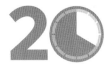

Tuna and Sweetcorn Wraps

Serves 4

2 eggs

400 g (13 oz) can tuna, drained

75 g (3 oz) canned sweetcorn, drained, or frozen sweetcorn

4 tablespoons mayonnaise

4 wholemeal flour tortillas or thin chapattis

1 tub cress, cut

4 pinches of paprika

pepper

- Place the eggs in a saucepan of water and bring to the boil. Reduce the heat and simmer for 10 minutes until hard-boiled. Remove from the pan and plunge into cold water to cool.

- Meanwhile, place the tuna and sweetcorn in a mixing bowl and season with pepper. Add the mayonnaise and mix together.

- Lay the tortillas or chapattis on a chopping board and divide the tuna mixture between them, piled across the middle of each. Shell the eggs and roughly chop, then scatter over the tuna mixture. Scatter with the cress. Sprinkle each with a pinch of paprika, then roll up tightly and cut in half to serve. Wrap in greaseproof paper to travel, if liked.

 Tuna and Cress Dip with Crudités and Crispy Tortillas Cut 2 flour tortillas into triangles and dry-fry in a frying pan for 1 minute on each side until slightly crisp. Remove and set aside to cool. Place a 200 g (7 oz) can tuna, drained and 100 g (3½ oz) canned sweetcorn, drained, or frozen sweetcorn in a bowl with 4 tablespoons mayonnaise and mix well. Season with pepper, then stir in a tub of snipped cress and mix well. Transfer to a serving bowl and serve with sugarsnap peas and the tortillas.

 Baked Tuna and Sweetcorn Tortillas Mix a 400 g (13 oz) can tuna, drained, in a bowl with 100 g (3½ oz) grated Cheddar cheese, 100 g (3½ oz) canned sweetcorn, drained, or frozen sweetcorn and 4 roughly chopped spring onions. Lay 4 flour tortillas on a chopping board and divide the tuna mixture between them, piling on to a quarter of the area of each. Fold the tortillas into quarters to enclose the filling. Arrange in a single layer in an ovenproof dish and scatter with a further 75 g (3 oz) grated Cheddar cheese. Cook under a preheated medium grill for 5–7 minutes until the cheese has melted and the tortillas are piping hot. Serve with salad, if liked.

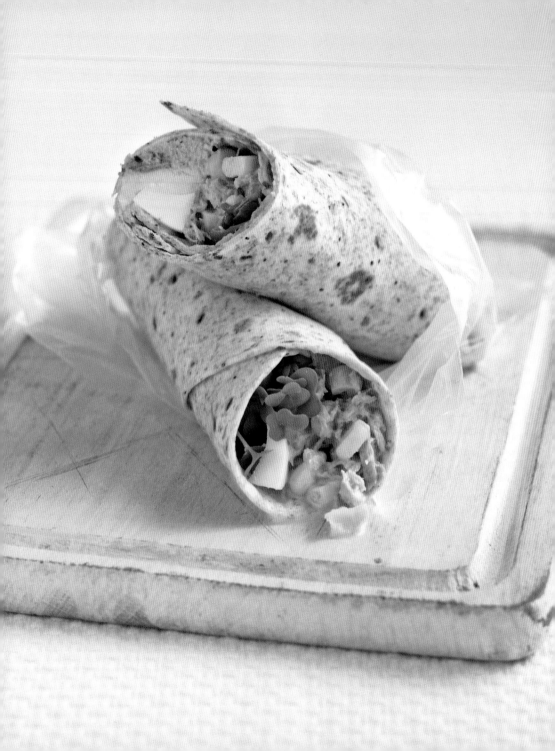

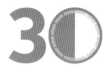

Wholemeal Cheese Straws with Pesto Dip

Serves 4

50 g (2 oz) softened butter, plus extra for greasing

125 g (4 oz) Cheddar cheese, grated

125 g (4 oz) wholemeal plain flour, plus extra for dusting

beaten egg, to glaze

2 tablespoons sesame seeds

¼ teaspoon chilli powder

For the dip

3 tablespoons pesto

75 g (3 oz) soft cheese

3 tablespoons milk

- Lightly grease a baking sheet.

- Blend the butter and cheese in a food processor. Stir in the flour and 3 tbsp water and form into a soft dough. Turn out onto a lightly floured surface and roll out to about 0.5 cm (¼ inch) thick. Brush with beaten egg, then cut into 1.5 cm (¾ inch) x 10 cm long strips and sprinkle with the sesame seeds and chilli powder. Place on the prepared baking sheet and bake in a preheated oven, 200°C (400°F), Gas Mark 6, for 10–15 minutes until crisp.

- Meanwhile, make the dip. Mix the pesto with the soft cheese and milk. Place in a small dipping bowl to serve with the warm cheese straws.

 Cheese Straws with Cheesy Basil and Pine Nut Dip Put 200 g (7 oz) soft cheese into a bowl with 3 tablespoons milk and blend until smooth. Roughly chop a handful of basil and add to the cheese along with 3 tablespoons grated Parmesan cheese and 2 tablespoons roughly chopped pine nuts. Season generously with pepper and serve with ready-made cheese straws.

 Pesto and Cheese Squares Unroll 375 g (12 oz) ready-rolled shortcrust pastry on a chopping board and spread with 4 tablespoons pesto, right to the edges. Cut into 15 squares (5 x 3) and place on a baking sheet, spaced apart. Finely grate 50 g (2 oz) Parmesan cheese and scatter over the top of each, along with 1 tablespoon sesame seeds and 1 tablespoon pumpkin seeds. Bake in a preheated oven, 220°C (425°F), Gas Mark 7, for 10–12 minutes until golden and cooked through. Serve warm.

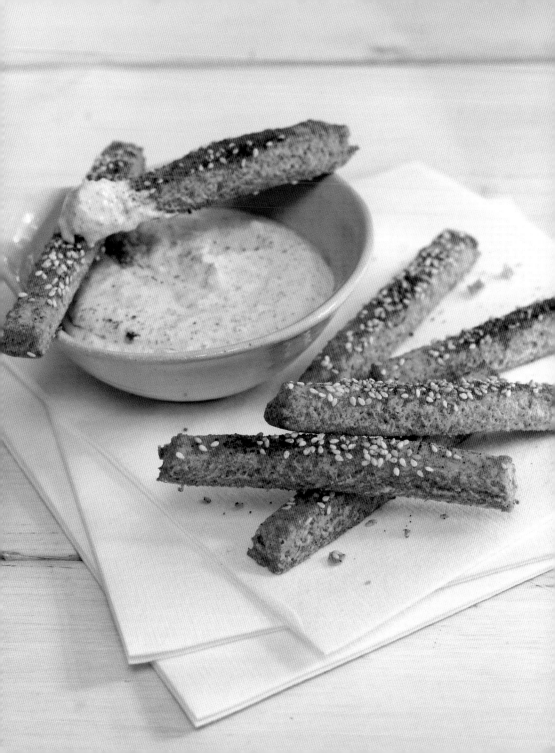

3 **0** Picnic Loaf

Serves 6

1 medium cottage loaf
125 g (4 oz) salami
125 g (4 oz) sliced turkey
handful of basil leaves
3 tomatoes, sliced
150 g (5 oz) mozzarella cheese,
  drained and sliced
1 small red onion, cut into rings
2 handfuls of rocket leaves
75 g (3 oz) pitted black olives
75 g (3 oz) Cheddar cheese, thinly
  sliced

- Cut the top off the loaf, about 3.5 cm (1½ inches) down from the top, and hollow out the inside of the loaf, pulling the soft bread out with your hands and leaving about a 2.5 cm (1 inch) edge.

- Start by layering the salami into the base of the hollowed-out loaf, then cover with the turkey slices. Place a layer of basil leaves on top of the turkey, then layer the tomato and mozzarella slices. Cover with the red onion rings and scatter over the rocket leaves. Top with the olives and finish with a layer of the Cheddar. Place the cottage loaf top back on and press down firmly.

- Wrap in greaseproof paper and refrigerate until needed. Cut into wedges to serve.

---

1 **0** **Mini Picnic Rolls**
Cut 2 crusty rolls a in half horizontally. Pull out the soft bread from the base of each and fill with 2 slices of wafer-thin ham, 2 slices of mozzarella cheese, 3 slices of tomato and 4 slices of cucumber. Lightly spread the top of each with 1 teaspoon mayonnaise, then place the top of the roll back on the base. Press down well, cut in half and secure with a cocktail stick if necessary. Serve half a well-filled roll per child.

2 **0** **Warm Ciabatta Picnic Loaf**
Cut 1 ciabatta loaf horizontally about one-third of the way down. Pull out half of the soft bread from the base of the loaf. Drain a 400 g (13 oz) jar of roasted peppers and place in the base of the ciabatta in layers with 150 g (5 oz) drained and sliced mozzarella cheese and 50 g (2 oz) salami. Place on a baking sheet, put the top back on and secure with cocktail sticks. Place in a preheated oven,

200°C (400°F), Gas Mark 6, for 5–10 minutes to warm through. Serve in chunky slices.

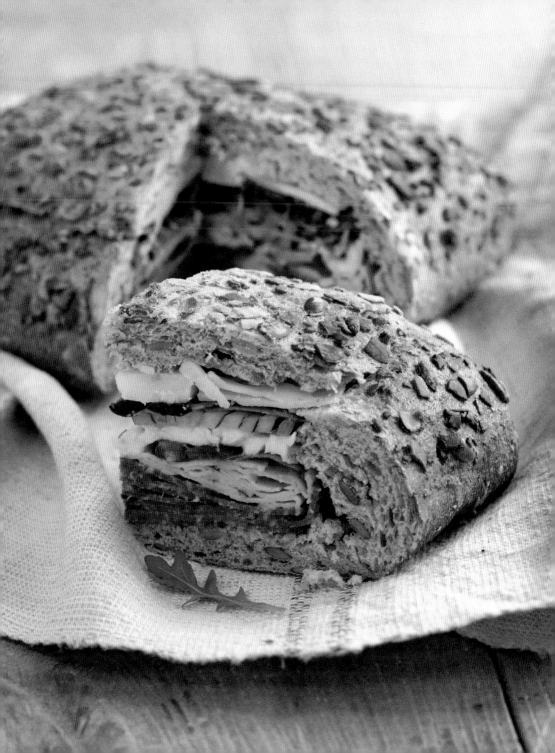

30 Crunchy Chicken Pesto Dippers

Serves 4

150 ml (¼ pint) ready-made
pesto
500 g (1 lb) boneless, skinless
chicken breast, cut into chunks
or thick slices
175 g (6 oz) couscous
3 tablespoons crème fraîche
crudités, such as red pepper and
carrot sticks, to serve (optional)

- Place 1 tablespoon of the pesto in a small bowl and reserve. Put the remaining pesto in a mixing bowl with the chicken and toss well to coat the chicken.

- Put the couscous in a bowl. Lightly coat the chicken, one piece at a time, in the couscous, then place on a baking sheet, spaced apart. Bake in a preheated oven, 200 °C (400 °F), Gas Mark 6, for 20–25 minutes, until the chicken is tender and cooked through and the outer coating is golden.

- Meanwhile, mix the crème fraîche with the reserved pesto and place in a small bowl on a serving platter with the crudités. Using tongs, transfer the crunchy pesto chicken on to the serving platter. Serve while warm, with cocktail stick flags, for kids to share.

---

10 **Chicken Skewers with Warm Pesto Dip** Heat 5 tablespoons olive oil in a frying pan and cook 4 tablespoons pine nuts for 2 minutes until golden. Place 4 tablespoons grated Parmesan cheese in a food processor with 2 x 30 g (1¼ oz) packets of basil leaves, pour over the hot oil and pine nuts and whizz until smooth. Add 3 tablespoons ricotta cheese and whizz again. Pour into a small heatproof serving dish and serve with freshly cut crudités and shop-bought chicken skewers or mini-fillets for dipping.

20 **Pesto Chicken Couscous** Place a 110 g (3¾ oz) packet of flavoured couscous in a bowl. Pour over enough hot water to cover, according to the packet instructions, and set aside to swell for 15 minutes. Meanwhile, cut 450 g (14½ oz) boneless, skinless chicken breasts into chunks and toss with 4 tablespoons pesto to coat. Place the chunks on a foil-lined grill rack and cook under a preheated grill for 10–12 minutes, turning once, until golden and cooked through. Toss into the couscous along with 2 tablespoons toasted pine nuts and a handful of chopped basil leaves.

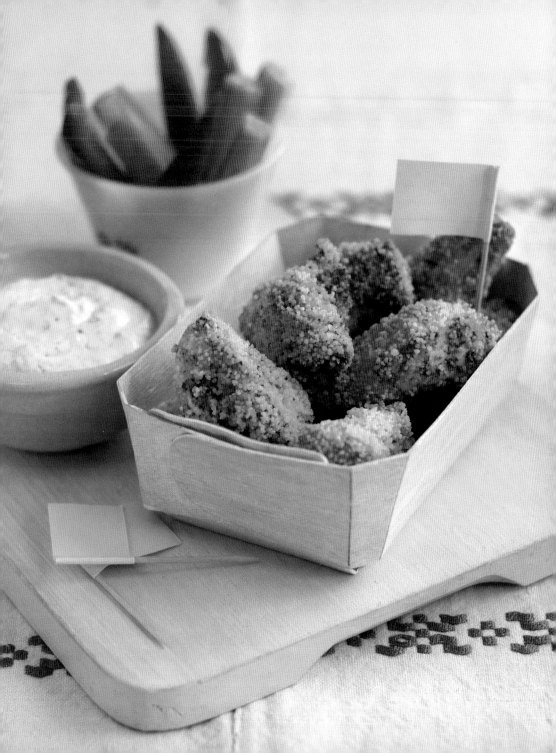

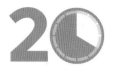

Brown Rice Salad with Peanuts and Raisins

Serves 4

200 g (7 oz) easy-cook brown rice

bunch of spring onions, roughly chopped

125 g (4 oz) raisins

1 red pepper, cored, deseeded and sliced

75 g (3 oz) roasted peanuts

2 tablespoons dark soy sauce

1 tablespoon sesame oil

- Cook the rice in a saucepan of lightly salted boiling water for 15–18 minutes until tender.

- Meanwhile, place the spring onions, raisins, red pepper and peanuts in a large bowl and toss with the soy sauce and sesame oil until well coated.

- Once the rice is cooked, drain it in a sieve and rinse with cold water until cold. Once cold and drained, add to the other ingredients and toss well to coat and mix.

- Turn into a serving bowl and serve, or place in a lunch box with slices of cheese or meat to serve alongside, if liked.

 ### Speedy Raisin and Peanut Rice Salad

Place 250 g (8 oz) ready-cooked fresh rice in a bowl with 125 g (4 oz) raisins and 2 large peeled and grated carrots and 6 tablespoons chopped parsley. Tip in 50 g (2 oz) roughly chopped peanuts and toss well.

 ### Fruit and Nut Pilaf Rice

Cook 250 g (8 oz) easy-cook brown rice in a large saucepan of lightly salted boiling water for 15–18 minutes until tender. Meanwhile, heat 3 tablespoons olive oil in a frying pan over a high heat and cook 1 sliced red onion and 1 small cored, deseeded and sliced red pepper for 4–5 minutes until soft. Add 75 g (3 oz) pine nuts and 1 bunch of roughly chopped spring onions and cook for a further 2–3 minutes until the pine nuts are golden. Once the rice is cooked, drain well. Add the hot rice to the pan with the peppers and pine nuts and toss well. Add 125 g (4 oz) raisins and 75 g (3 oz) chopped ready-to-eat dried apricots. Toss well, then add 4 tablespoons chopped parsley and serve hot.

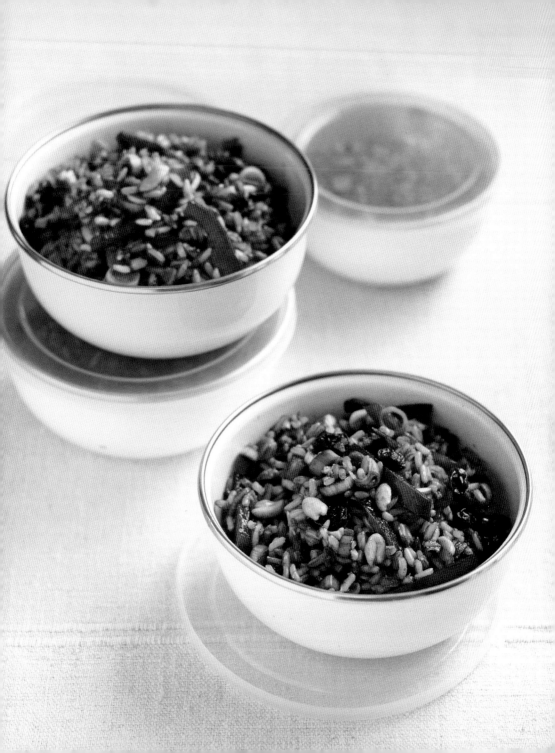

30 Ricotta and Tomato Scones

Makes 8

500 g (1 lb) self-raising flour, plus extra for dusting

250 g (8 oz) ricotta cheese, plus extra to serve (optional)

1 egg

250 ml (8 fl oz) milk

3 tablespoons chopped mixed herbs, such as basil, parsley and oregano

4 sun-dried tomatoes, drained and roughly chopped

milk, to glaze

1 tablespoon sesame seeds

salt and pepper

butter, to serve (optional)

- Sift the flour into a food processor and season with a little salt and pepper. Place the ricotta, egg, milk, herbs and tomatoes in a separate bowl and beat together well. Add the ricotta mixture to the flour and whizz to form a soft dough. Turn out on to a lightly floured surface and roll out to about 2.5 cm (1 inch) thick.

- Stamp out 8 scones using a 6 cm (2½ inch) cutter and place on a baking sheet. Brush with a little milk and scatter with sesame seeds. Bake in a preheated oven, 200°C (400°F), Gas Mark 6, for 15 minutes until golden and risen.

- Serve warm with butter or extra ricotta for spreading.

 Quick Ricotta and Tomato-Topped Scones Cut 4 ready-made cheese scones in half. Mix 250 g (8 oz) ricotta cheese with 5 roughly chopped sun-dried tomatoes and 4 tablespoons chopped basil. Spread spoonfuls of the mixture on each of the scone halves, top with 2 pitted black olives and serve with extra basil leaves to garnish, if liked. The scones can be warmed in a preheated oven, 200°C (400°F), Gas Mark 6, for 5 minutes while making the ricotta topping, if preferred.

 Scone Wedges with Ricotta and Tomato Topping Make up a 320 g (11 oz) packet scone mix according to the packet instructions using egg and milk. Roll out into a rough round and cut into 8 wedges. Place the wedges, spaced well apart, on a baking sheet and brush with milk. Sprinkle with 1 tablespoon sesame seeds and bake in a preheated oven, 230°C (450°F), Gas Mark 8, for 10–12 minutes until golden. Meanwhile, mix 250 g (8 oz) ricotta cheese with 5 roughly chopped sun-dried tomatoes and 4 tablespoons basil leaves in a bowl. To serve, cut open the warm scones and spread with the herb and tomato ricotta mixture.

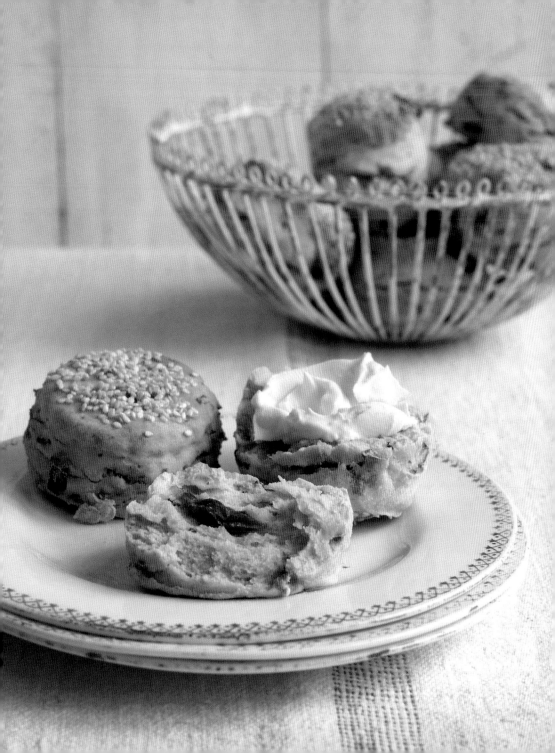

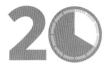

Honeyed Duck Strips in Lettuce 'Boats'

Serves 4

2 tablespoons sesame oil

2 duck breasts, about 175 g (6 oz) each, cut into thin strips

2 teaspoons Chinese five spice powder

2 tablespoons dark soy sauce

2 tablespoons clear honey

2 tablespoons toasted sesame seeds

8 Little Gem lettuce leaves

To garnish

4 spring onions, finely chopped

1 small carrot, peeled and grated

crusty bread, to serve (optional)

- Heat the oil in a heavy-based frying pan. Toss the duck strips with the Chinese five spice powder in a bowl, then fry over a high heat for 8–10 minutes until cooked and crispy. Add the soy sauce and honey and cook for a further 2 minutes to coat in the sticky glaze. Scatter with the sesame seeds and keep warm.

- Wash and pat dry the lettuce leaves and place on a serving board. Place spoonfuls of the duck into the leaves, then garnish each with the spring onions and carrot.

- Serve with crusty bread, if liked.

 Honeyed Duck Stir-Fry

Heat 2 tablespoons sesame oil in a large heavy-based frying pan and cook 175 g (6 oz) very thinly sliced duck breast over a high heat for 4 minutes. Add 500 g (1 lb) ready-prepared 'family stir-fry' vegetables to the pan with 2 teaspoons Chinese five spice powder and stir-fry for 3–4 minutes until tender but still retaining their shape. Add 1 tablespoon clear honey, 2 tablespoons sesame seeds and 2 tablespoons soy sauce and stir-fry for 2 minutes, then serve in warmed bowls.

 Honey Duck Pilaf

Cook 250 g (8 oz) easy-cook white or easy-cook basmati rice in a large saucepan of lightly salted boiling water for 15 minutes until tender. Meanwhile, heat 2 tablespoons sesame oil in a large heavy-based frying pan and cook 2 very thinly sliced duck breasts, about 175 g (6 oz) each, over a high heat for 5 minutes until beginning to turn golden. Add 2 teaspoons Chinese five spice powder and cook for a further 3–4 minutes. Add 4 finely shredded spring onions and 1 large peeled and finely shredded carrot and cook over a high heat for 2 minutes. Add 1 tablespoon dark soy sauce and 2 tablespoons clear honey, increase the heat and cook for a further 2 minutes. Drain the rice, then add to the duck mixture and stir for 2 minutes. Serve sprinkled with chopped coriander, if liked.

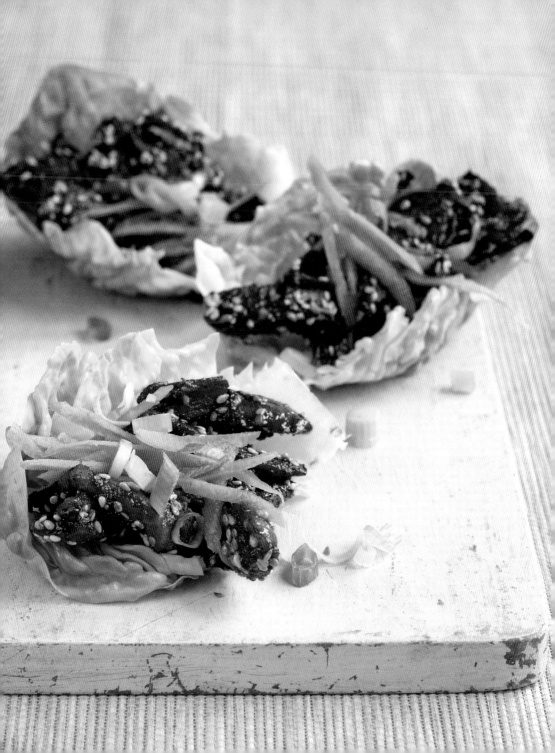

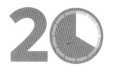

Pineapple and Chunky Ham Skewers

Serves 4

500 g (1 lb) bacon or gammon
   piece
2 tablespoons olive oil
1 teaspoon wholegrain mustard
2 tablespoons clear honey
1 tablespoon chopped parsley
½ pineapple, peeled, cored and
   cut into 16 chunks
crudites, to serve (optional)

- Cut the bacon or gammon into 24 chunky pieces. Heat 1 tablespoon of the oil in a heavy-based frying pan and cook the bacon or gammon pieces over a medium-high heat for 5–7 minutes until cooked through and golden in places. Add the honey and parsley and toss to coat the ham pieces. Keep warm.

- In a separate frying pan, heat the remaining oil and cook the pineapple chunks over a high heat for 4–5 minutes until golden and hot.

- Thread 3 chunks of ham and 2 chunks of pineapple on to 8 small bamboo skewers and serve with crudites.

 Warm Ham and Pineapple Pittas

Lightly toast 4 pittas and keep warm. Heat 125 g (4 oz) butter in a frying pan and cook a 200 g (7 oz) can pineapple cubes, drained over a high heat for 5 minutes until piping hot and golden in places. Add 175 g (6 oz) ham offcuts and cook for a further 3 minutes until beginning to turn golden in places. Mix 2 tablespoons clear honey with 1 teaspoon wholegrain mustard and toss into the pan. Load into the pittas and serve with salad, if liked.

 Pineapple and Ham Stir-Fry

Heat 2 tablespoons olive oil in a wok or frying pan and cook a 375 g (12 oz) bacon or gammon piece, cut into 2.5 cm (1 inch) cubes, for 10 minutes until golden and cooked through. Add ½ pineapple, peeled and cut into chunks, and stir-fry over a high heat for a further 5 minutes until the pineapple is beginning to turn golden. Core, deseed and cut 1 red and 1 green pepper into chunks, add to the pan and stir-fry for 3–4 minutes until beginning to soften. Mix 1 tablespoon wholegrain mustard with 3 tablespoons clear honey and 3 tablespoons chopped parsley, pour into the pan and cook, stirring and tossing, for a further 2–3 minutes until the gammon and pineapple are coated in the mustard glaze. Serve with egg noodles.

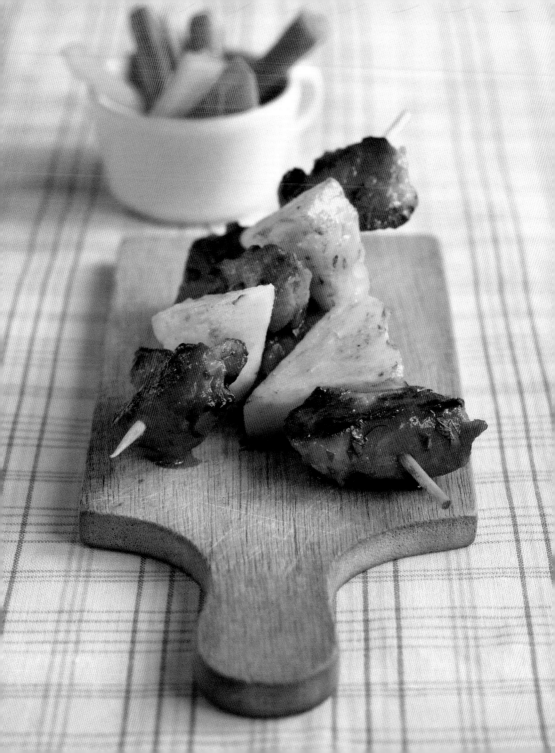

Mini Brie and Tomato Quiches

Serves 4

175 g (6 oz) ready-rolled
  shortcrust pastry
16 cherry tomatoes
175 g (6 oz) Brie, cut into cubes
1 tablespoon chopped parsley
2 eggs
2 tablespoons crème fraîche
pepper
salad or baked beans, to serve
  (optional)

- Unroll the pastry and cut into 4 x 12 cm (5 inch) squares. Use to line a 4-hole Yorkshire pudding tin and press down. Put 4 tomatoes in each and divide the Brie between them. Mix together the parsley, eggs and crème fraîche, beating until smooth, and season with a little pepper. Pour into the pastry cases to just cover the cheese.

- Bake in a preheated oven, 200°C (400°F), Gas Mark 6, for 20 minutes until golden and puffed, and the pastry is cooked.

- Serve hot with a simple salad or baked beans, if liked.

Brie and Tomato Crostini

Cut a ciabatta loaf in half both horizontally and lengthways to make 4 pieces. Drizzle each with 1 tablespoon olive oil and place on a baking sheet. Cook under a preheated hot grill for 1 minute until beginning to toast. Remove and load each with 50 g (2 oz) Brie slices and 6 cherry tomatoes. Season generously with pepper. Grill for a further 4–5 minutes until the tomatoes split slightly and the Brie melts and turns golden, then serve.

Brie and Tomato Pots

Divide 12 cherry tomatoes between 4 ramekins. Cut 175 g (6 oz) Brie into chunks, then divide between the ramekins. Beat 4 eggs with 1 tablespoon chopped parsley and 2 tablespoons crème fraîche and season generously with pepper. Pour over the tomatoes and Brie in the ramekins, then place on a baking sheet and bake in a preheated oven, 220°C (425°F), Gas Mark 7, for 15 minutes until well puffed up and turning pale golden. Leave to cool slightly, then serve on small plates with crusty bread.

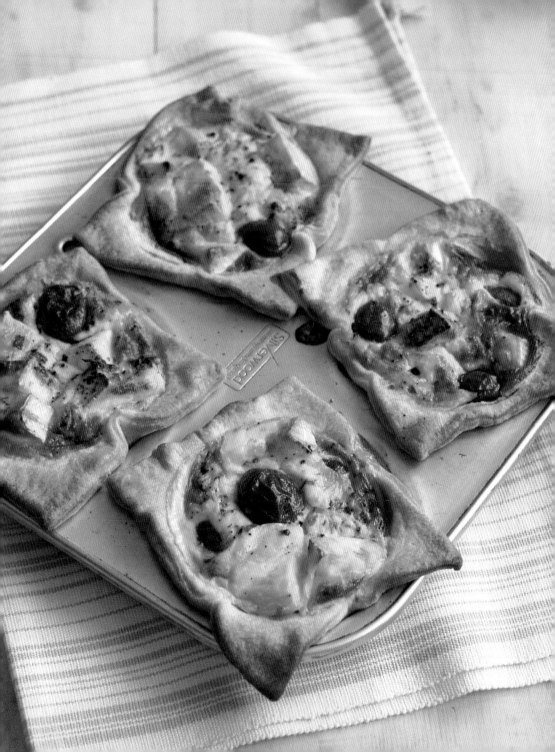

30 Curried Chicken Couscous Salad

Serves 4

125 g (4 oz) barley couscous

3 tablespoons olive oil

1 red onion, sliced

375 g (12 oz) boneless, skinless chicken breast, thinly sliced

bunch of spring onions, cut into strips

4 tablespoons korma curry paste

2 tablespoons water

1 ripe mango, peeled, stoned and cut into chunks

4 tablespoons chopped coriander (optional)

natural yogurt, to serve (optional)

- Place the couscous in a bowl and pour over enough lightly salted water to just cover. Set aside for 20 minutes to swell.

- Meanwhile, heat the oil in a frying pan and cook the red onion and chicken slices over a high heat for 5 minutes, then reduce the heat, add the spring onions and cook for a further 3–4 minutes until softened and cooked through. Keep warm.

- In a separate frying pan, heat the curry paste over a low heat until softened, adding the measurement water to loosen. Drain the couscous and transfer to the pan with the curry paste and toss and stir to coat and heat, for about 2 minutes.

- Toss the chicken and onions into the curried couscous with the mango and coriander, if using, and toss again before serving with spoonfuls of natural yogurt, if liked.

 Curried Chicken and Mint Couscous

Thinly slice 250 g (8 oz) boneless, skinless chicken breasts. Heat 3 tablespoons olive oil in a large heavy-based frying pan and cook the chicken over a high heat for 5 minutes until golden and cooked through. Add 2 tablespoons korma curry paste with 2 tablespoons water and heat for 2 minutes until piping hot. Transfer to a mixing bowl. Add 2 x 300 g (10 oz) tubs tomato and cucumber couscous salad and toss into the chicken with 2 tablespoons chopped mint. Serve with spoonfuls of tzatziki.

 Curried Chicken Salad with

Couscous Place a 110 g (3¾ oz) packet flavoured couscous in a bowl. Pour over hot water according to the packet instructions and set aside to swell. Meanwhile, place 6 tablespoons mayonnaise in a bowl with 4 tablespoons natural yogurt and 3 tablespoons korma curry paste and mix together. Add 375 g (12 oz) shop-bought ready-cooked chicken, 5 roughly chopped spring onions, 1 small peeled, stoned and roughly chopped mango and 4 tablespoons chopped coriander.

Stir well to coat in the curried mayonnaise and serve alongside the couscous.

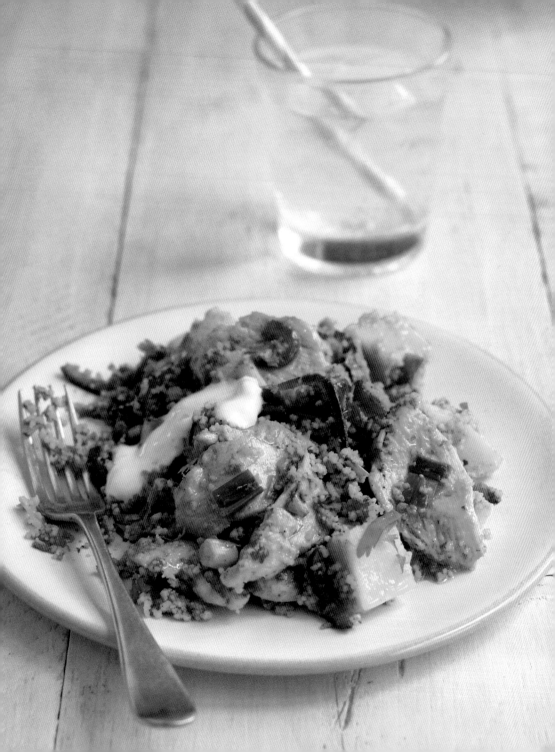

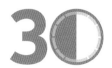 # Vegetable and Cheese Pasties

Makes 4

500 g (1 lb) pack shortcrust
pastry
flour, for dusting
25 g (1 oz) butter, melted
400 g (13 oz) ready-prepared
vegetable casserole mix
(carrots, swede, turnip and
potato cubes), roughly chopped
into about 1 cm (½ inch) cubes
if too large
125 g (4 oz) mature Cheddar
cheese, grated
1 tablespoon dried thyme
beaten egg, to glaze
pepper

- Roll out the pastry on a lightly floured surface and cut out 4 x 25 cm (10 inch) circles, using a plate if necessary.

- Put the melted butter and oil in a bowl with the vegetables and toss well. Season with plenty of pepper and toss again. Add the cheese and thyme and toss well. Divide the vegetable and cheese mixture between the 4 circles of pastry. Dampen the rims of the pastry using a brush and a little water, then lift the pastry edges up and over the filling to meet one another and pinch together to hold in a pasty shape. Place on a large baking sheet and crimp the edges using your fingers.

- Brush with beaten egg and bake in a preheated oven, 200°C (400°F), Gas Mark 6, for 20 minutes until golden and cooked through. The vegetables cook in their own steam inside the pastry and should be tender.

 Cheesy Vegetable Soup

Place 400 g (13 oz) ready-prepared vegetable casserole mix in a saucepan with 600 ml (1 pint) vegetable stock and bring to the boil. Cover, reduce the heat and simmer for 8 minutes, then transfer to a food processor with 75 g (3 oz) grated Cheddar cheese, 2 tablespoons thyme leaves and 1 teaspoon Dijon mustard and whizz until smooth and thick. Divide between 2 bowls and serve with warm crusty bread.

 Carrot and Cheese Tarts

Unroll 300 g (10 oz) ready-rolled shortcrust pastry, stamp out 4 x 12 cm (5 inch) circles and use to line a 4-hole Yorkshire pudding tin. Bake in a preheated oven, 200°C (400°F), Gas Mark 6, for 10 minutes until pale golden. Meanwhile, scatter 2 large peeled and roughly chopped carrots in a roasting tin and toss with 3 tablespoons olive oil. Roast at the top of the oven above the pastry tart cases for 12 minutes until lightly charred in places and tender. Meanwhile, cut 125 g (4 oz) Cheddar cheese into small cubes and place in a bowl with 1 tablespoon olive oil and 1 tablespoon chopped thyme. Add the roasted carrots to the bowl and toss to warm and slightly melt the cheese. Divide the filling between the tarts and serve warm.

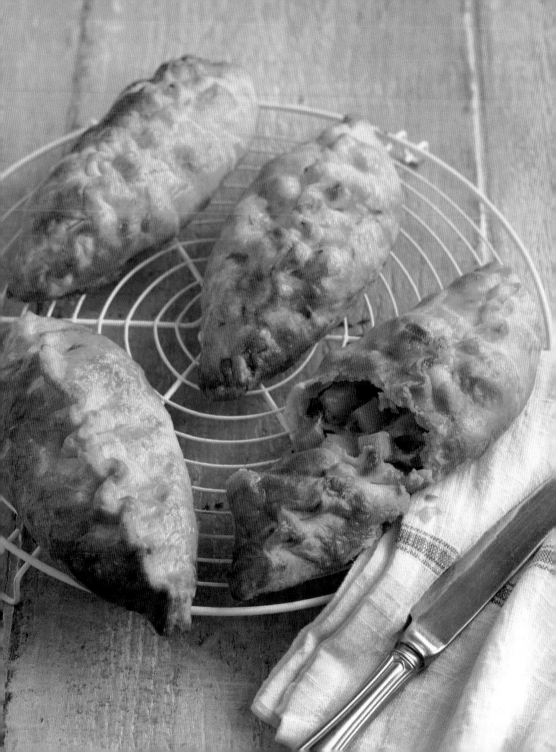

30 Sweet and Sticky Chicken Drumsticks with Coleslaw

Serves 4

2 tablespoons clear honey
1 tablespoon wholegrain mustard
3 tablespoons tomato ketchup
2 teaspoons dark soy sauce
1 tablespoon olive oil
8 chicken drumsticks

For the coleslaw

¼ small savoy cabbage, shredded
2 large carrots, peeled and
    roughly grated
2 tablespoons chopped parsley
5 tablespoons mayonnaise
4 tablespoons crème fraîche
1 tablespoon water
pepper
bread rolls, to serve (optional)

- Place the honey, mustard seeds, ketchup, soy sauce and oil in a large mixing bowl and blend well. Add the chicken drumsticks and toss in the marinade. Place in a roasting tin, brush over any remaining marinade and cook in a preheated oven, 220°C (425°F), Gas Mark 7, for 20–25 minutes until golden and cooked through.

- Meanwhile, make the coleslaw. Place the shredded cabbage, carrots and parsley in a mixing bowl and toss together. Mix together the mayonnaise, crème fraîche and measurement water in a separate bowl then season well with pepper. Spoon over the coleslaw, then mix and toss well to coat in the dressing.

- Serve the chicken drumsticks with the coleslaw and bread rolls, if liked.

---

1 Chicken Coleslaw Pitta Breads

Shred ¼ white or savoy cabbage and place in a bowl with 2 peeled and grated carrots. Toss in 2 tablespoons chopped parsley. Tear 250 g (8 oz) shop-bought ready-cooked chicken into shreds and add to the coleslaw mix. Add 3 tablespoons raisins. Mix 5 tablespoons mayonnaise with 2 tablespoons water, stir into the chicken coleslaw and mix to coat. Pile into warm toasted pittas for a great tea!

2 Sticky Chicken Skewers with Red Coleslaw Slice 250 g (8 oz) boneless, skinless chicken breast into long, thin slices. Place 2 tablespoons clear honey, 1 tablespoon wholegrain mustard, 3 tablespoons tomato ketchup, 2 teaspoons dark soy sauce and 1 tablespoon olive oil in a bowl and mix well. Add the chicken strips and toss well. Thread on to 4 wooden or metal skewers, then cook under a preheated medium grill for 10 minutes, turning occasionally, until golden and cooked through. Meanwhile, to make the red coleslaw, place ¼ small shredded red cabbage in a bowl with 1 large peeled and grated carrot and 5 tablespoons mayonnaise mixed with 3 tablespoons water. Toss well to coat in the dressing. Serve the skewers with the coleslaw and bread rolls, if liked.

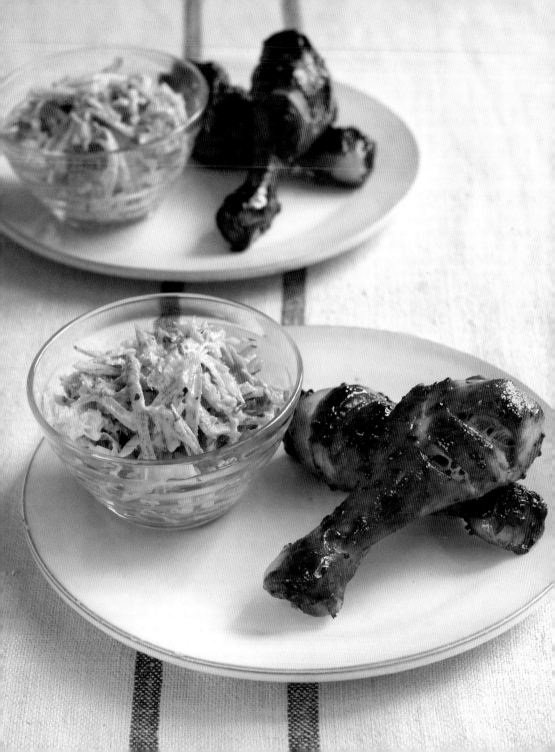

30 Mini Falafel Burgers

Serves 4

2 tablespoons sunflower oil
1 small onion, finely chopped
1 garlic clove, crushed
400 g (13 oz) can chickpeas,
  rinsed and drained
1 teaspoon ground cumin
1 teaspoon ground coriander
3 tablespoons chopped coriander
1 egg yolk
4 tablespoons natural yogurt
1 teaspoon mint sauce
salt and pepper

To serve

8 warm toasted mini pittas
salad leaves
8 cherry tomatoes, halved

- Heat 1 tablespoon of the oil in a large frying pan. Add the onion and cook over a low heat for 5 minutes until softened. Tip into a large mixing bowl with the chickpeas and ground spices and mash using a fork or potato masher until the chickpeas are broken down. Stir in the chopped coriander and season to taste. Add the egg yolk, then squish the mixture together with your hands.

- Mould the mixture into 8 small balls, then flatten into patty shapes. Heat the remaining oil in a frying pan and fry the falafels for 3 minutes on each side until golden brown and firm to the touch.

- Mix the yogurt with the mint sauce and spoon over the falafels (hot or cold). Serve with the mini pittas, salad leaves and tomatoes.

 Quick Chickpea and Spinach Stir-Fry

Heat 2 tablespoons oil in a pan and fry 1 roughly chopped onion for 2 minutes. Add a 400 g (13 oz) can chickpeas, rinsed and drained, and 300 g (10 oz) baby spinach leaves and cook for 2 minutes. Add ½ teaspoon ground cumin, ½ teaspoon ground coriander and ½ teaspoon minced garlic and cook for 2 minutes. Add 8 halved cherry tomatoes and cook for 1 minute. Pour in a 400 ml (14 fl oz) can coconut milk, heat for 2 minutes and serve with warm pitta bread.

 Chickpea and Coriander Dahl

Heat 2 tablespoons sunflower oil in a large frying pan and cook 1 small finely chopped onion and 1 crushed garlic clove for 3–4 minutes until softened. Add a 400 g (13 oz) can chickpeas, rinsed and drained, 1 teaspoon ground cumin, 1 teaspoon ground coriander and 3 tablespoons chopped coriander and cook for 2 minutes. Add 600 ml (1 pint) vegetable stock, bring to the boil and cook for 5 minutes. Transfer to a food processor and whizz until smooth. Make a raita by mixing 4 tablespoons natural yogurt with 1 teaspoon mint sauce and serve spooned over the dahl. Serve with warm naan breads cut into fingers for the kids to dip.

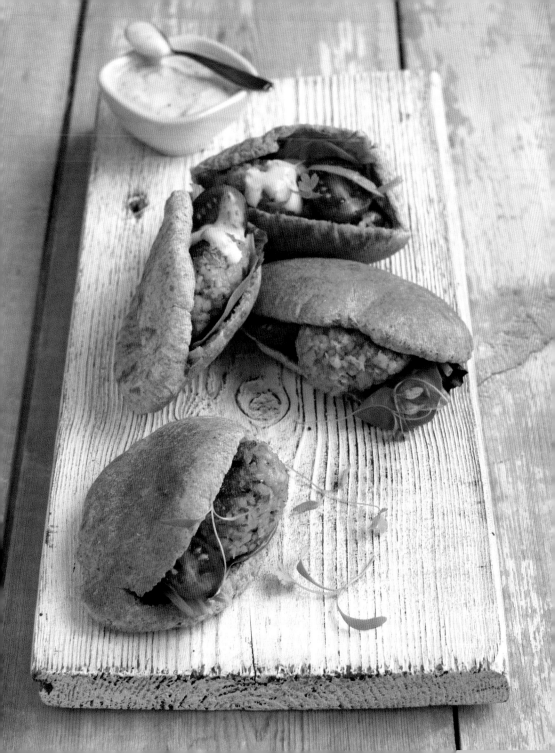

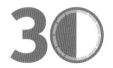

30 Marmite Pinwheels with Soft Cheese Dip

Makes 24

375 g (12 oz) ready-rolled puff pastry

2 tablespoons Marmite or other yeast extract

2 tablespoons chopped parsley, to garnish

For the soft cheese dip

200 g (7 oz) soft cheese

5 tablespoons milk

2 tablespoons chopped chives

1 tablespoon wholegrain mustard

pepper

- Unroll the pastry on a large chopping board. Spread thinly with the Marmite, right to the edges, then roll up tightly along its width. Using a sharp knife, cut the pastry into 24 slices and place well apart on a baking sheet. Bake in a preheated oven, 220°C (425°F), Gas Mark 7, for 15–18 minutes until golden and puffed.

- Meanwhile, make the soft cheese dip. Place the soft cheese in a bowl with the milk and chives. Season generously with pepper, add the mustard and mash well. Place in a small bowl and serve alongside the warm pinwheels.

1 Marmite and Cheese Toasties

Spread one side of 2 slices of brown or white bread with a little butter, then with ½ teaspoon Marmite. Layer the other piece of bread with 50 g (2 oz) thinly sliced Cheddar cheese and top with the Marmite slice, face down. Heat 15 g (½ oz) butter in a large frying pan and cook the sandwich over a high heat for 1 minute until golden, then turn the sandwich over and cook for a further 1 minute. Remove from the pan and cut into triangles to serve. Repeat to make 4 toasties.

2 Marmite and Cheese Open Tarts

Unroll 250 g (8 oz) ready-rolled puff pastry, cut into 4 equal rectangles and place on a baking sheet. Bake in a preheated oven, 220°C (425°F), Gas Mark 7, for 10–12 minutes until golden and puffed. Meanwhile, grate 75 g (3 oz) double Gloucester and 75 g (3 oz) Cheddar cheese and toss with 1 tablespoon chopped parsley. Remove the pastry from the oven, press down the centres and spread each with ½ teaspoon Marmite. Scatter with the cheese mixture and parsley and return to the oven for 5 minutes until melted. Serve with cherry tomatoes, if liked.

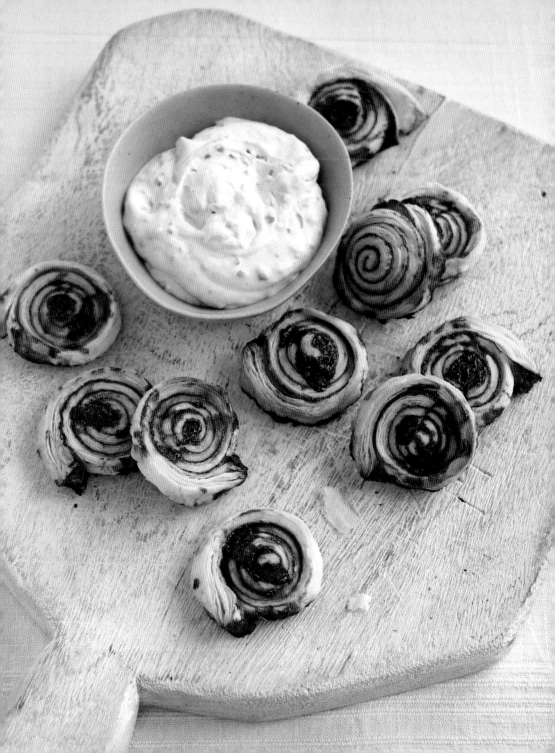

30 Pepperoni and Pepper Rolls

Makes 8

2 x 145 g (5 oz) packets pizza
base mix
2 tablespoons chopped oregano
flour, for dusting
1 tablespoon olive oil
¼ small red pepper, cored,
deseeded and roughly sliced
¼ small yellow pepper, cored,
deseeded and roughly sliced
¼ small green pepper, roughly
sliced
50 g (2 oz) pepperoni slices,
roughly chopped
4 tablespoons grated Cheddar
cheese

- Place the pizza base mix in a bowl with the oregano, add warm water according to the packet instructions and mix to form a smooth dough. Turn out on to a lightly floured surface and knead until smooth.

- Heat the oil in a heavy-based frying pan and cook the peppers over a medium heat for 4–5 minutes until soft, then add the pepperoni and cook for a further minute.

- Divide the dough into 8 pieces and make a well in the centre of each. Divide the peppers and pepperoni between the dough pieces and very roughly knead through the dough. Shape each into a rough ball and place on a baking sheet.

- Sprinkle with the Cheddar and bake in a preheated oven, 220°C (425°F), Gas Mark 7, for 20 minutes until golden and cooked through – the base should sound hollow when tapped. Serve warm.

 Grilled Pepperoni Pizza-Style Rolls

Cut 2 ciabatta rolls in half and place on a foil-lined grill rack, cut side up. Cook under a preheated medium grill for 1 minute until the tops are golden and crisp. Top each with 1 tablespoon drained and sliced roasted pepper antipasti, 2 slices of pepperoni and a slice of mozzarella cheese. Grill for 3–4 minutes until melted and golden, and serve hot.

 Pepperoni and Pepper Pizzas

Make up 2 x 145 g (5 oz) packets pizza base mix according to the packet instructions and divide the dough into 4 pieces. Roll out each piece to a very rough circle, about 1 cm (½ inch) thick, and place well apart on 1–2 baking sheets. Drain a 400 g (13 oz) jar of roasted peppers in oil, then toss in a bowl with ½ teaspoon dried oregano and divide between the pizzas. Top each with 3 slices of pepperoni and 1 tablespoon grated Cheddar cheese. Bake in a preheated oven, 220°C (425°F), Gas Mark 7, for 10 minutes until golden, and serve hot.

KID-BREA-GAN

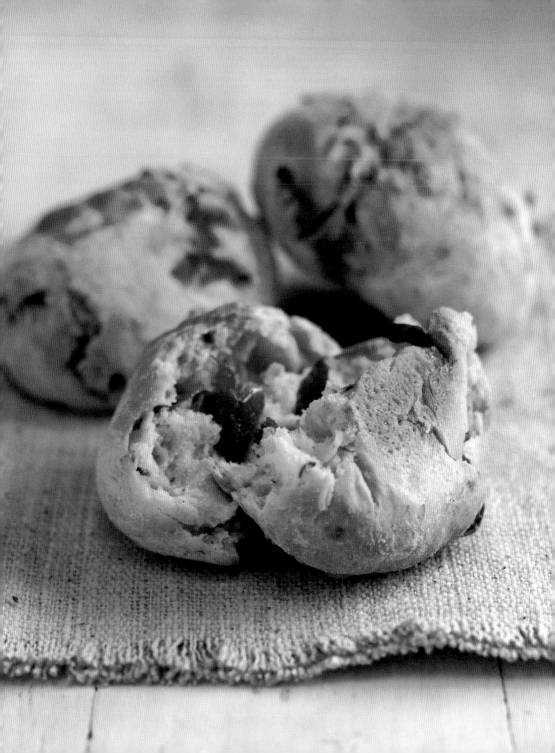

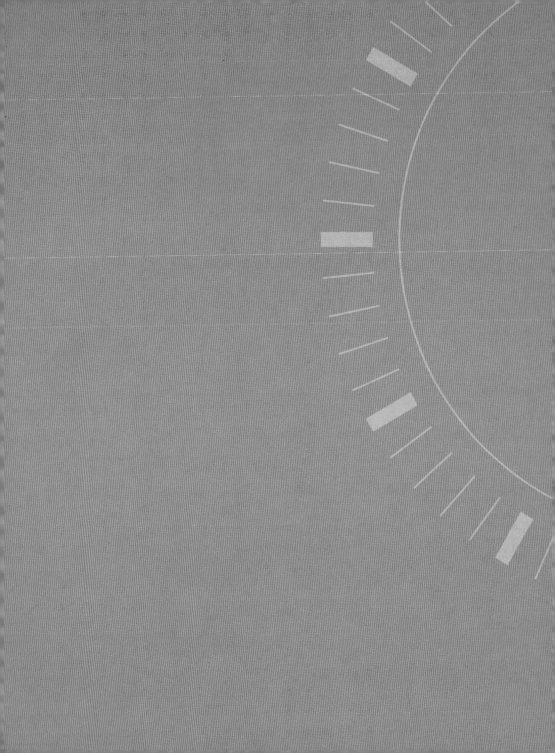

QuickCook

Kids' Favourites

Recipes listed by cooking time

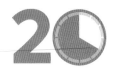

Pork and Apple Balls

Serves 4

1 small cox's apple, cored and grated (with skin on)

1 small onion, grated

250 g (8 oz) minced pork

50 g (2 oz) wholemeal breadcrumbs

3 tablespoons vegetable oil

To serve

tomato chutney

cherry tomato halves

- Place the apple and onion in a bowl with the pork and, using a fork, mash all the ingredients together well. Shape into 16 rough balls. Place the breadcrumbs on a plate and roll the balls in the breadcrumbs to lightly coat.

- Heat the oil in a large heavy-based frying pan and cook the balls over a medium-high heat for 8–10 minutes, turning frequently, until cooked through. Drain on kitchen paper.

- Serve warm with tomato chutney and cherry tomatoes, and provide bamboo paddle skewers for dipping the balls in the chutney.

 Pork Burgers with Apple Sauce

Put 300 g (10 oz) minced pork in a bowl and mix with 1 tablespoon wholegrain mustard and 2 tablespoons chopped parsley. Shape into 4 small, thin burgers. Heat 2 tablespoons oil in a frying pan and cook the burgers for 2–3 minutes on each side until golden and cooked through. Use to fill 4 wholemeal burger buns. Top with apple sauce and a small handful of salad leaves, if liked.

 Pork and Apple Shepherd's Pies

Heat 1 tablespoon olive oil in a pan and cook 250 g (8 oz) minced pork and 1 small chopped onion over a high heat for 5 minutes until beginning to turn golden. Add 1 small cored and chopped cox's apple (with skin on) and cook for a further 2–3 minutes, stirring continuously to help break up the pork. Add 300 ml (½ pint) chicken stock and 1 tablespoon Dijon mustard, stir into the pork and bring to the boil. Reduce the heat and simmer for 10 minutes. Remove from the heat and divide between 4 shallow ovenproof dishes. Stir in 25 g (1 oz) butter to 125 g (4 oz) chilled ready-made mashed potato and and season generously with pepper. Spoon the potato over the pork and apple filling and scatter each with 1 teaspoon grated Parmesan cheese. Cook under a preheated hot grill for 5–10 minutes until the top is golden and hot. Serve with peas or any green vegetable.

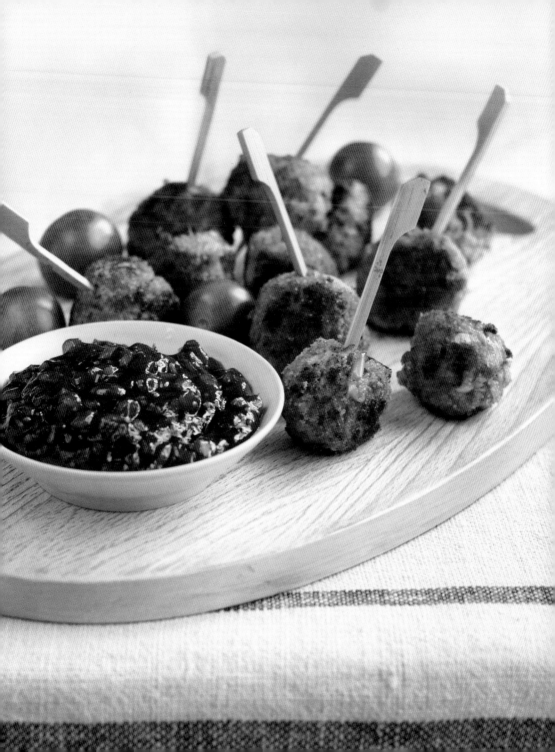

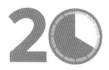 # Chicken and Sweetcorn Soup

Serves 4

1 tablespoon sunflower oil
1 boneless, skinless chicken breast
1 onion, chopped
500 ml (17 fl oz) chicken stock
150 ml (¼ pint) milk
1 large potato, cut into chunks
375 g (12 oz) canned sweetcorn, drained
salt and pepper
crispy bacon pieces, to garnish

- Heat the oil in a saucepan, add the whole chicken breast and the onion and fry over a low heat for about 5 minutes to soften but not colour. Add the stock, milk, potato and sweetcorn and bring to the boil. Reduce the heat, cover and simmer for 10 minutes until the potato and chicken are cooked through.

- Remove the chicken from the pan, place on a board and shred or chop. Blend the soup with a hand-held blender or in a food processor until almost smooth. Season with salt and pepper, return the chicken to the pan and reheat.

- Serve sprinkled with crispy bacon pieces.

 Chunky Chicken, Sweetcorn and Bacon Soup Dry-fry 3 chopped bacon rashers in a large saucepan. Stir in 600 ml (1 pint) ready-made creamy mushroom soup, 200 g (7 oz) cooked shredded chicken and a 200 g (7 oz) can sweetcorn, drained. Simmer for 2 minutes, adding a little water if the soup is too thick.

 Creamy Chicken, Sweetcorn and Bacon Casserole Heat 2 tablespoons olive oil in a large frying pan and fry 4 boneless, skinless chicken breasts for 5 minutes, turning once. Remove from the pan and set aside. Add 1 chopped onion to the pan with 3 chopped bacon rashers and 1 peeled and sliced carrot and fry for a further 5 minutes. Stir in 200 ml (7 fl oz) crème fraîche and crumble in a chicken stock cube. Heat, stirring, adding a little water if necessary to make a smooth sauce. Add a 200 g (7 oz) can sweetcorn, drained. Return the chicken to the pan, cover and simmer for 10 minutes until the chicken and vegetables are cooked through. Serve with mashed potato.

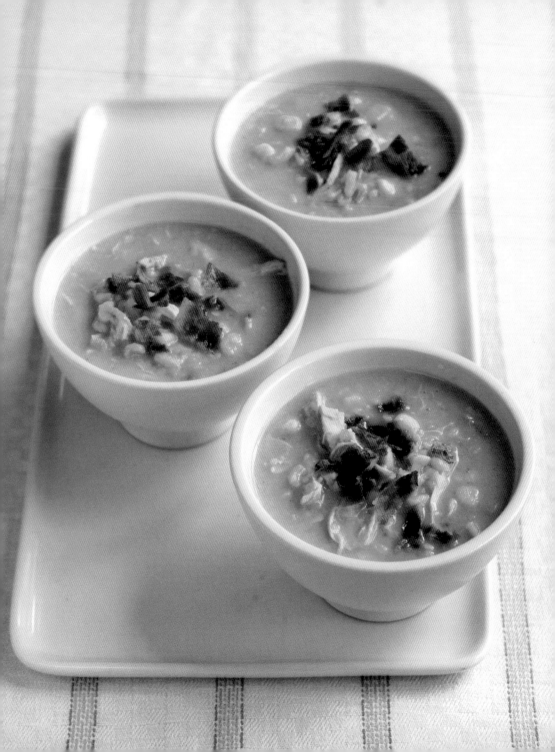

30 Corned Beef and Tomato Pies

Makes 4

1 tablespoon olive oil
1 small onion, finely chopped
325 g (11 oz) can corned beef
1 teaspoon Dijon mustard
8 cherry tomatoes, halved
2 tablespoons chopped parsley
375 g (12 oz) ready-rolled puff
   pastry
beaten egg, to glaze

- Heat the oil in a large heavy-based frying pan and cook the onion for 3–4 minutes until softened.

- Meanwhile, place the corned beef in a bowl, break it into chunks using a fork and mix with the mustard. Add to the pan with the onion and cook, gently stirring, for 2–3 minutes until warm, adding the cherry tomato halves for the final minute. Sprinkle over the parsley and gently toss.

- Cut the pastry into 4 x 12 cm (5 inch) squares and 4 x 10 cm (4 inch) squares (rolling the pastry a little wider first if necessary. Use the larger pieces to line a 4-hole Yorkshire pudding tin with the corners overlapping the hole edges.

- Divide the corned beef and tomato mixture between the pastry cases. Lightly brush the edges of each pie with water and place the smaller squares on top as lids. Press down well to adhere, and make a hole in the centre of each. Brush with beaten egg and bake in a preheated oven, 200°C (400°F), Gas Mark 6, for 20 minutes until golden and puffed. Serve.

 Corned Beef and Tomato Hash Pie

Heat 1 tablespoon oil in a frying pan. Add 350 g (11½ oz) canned mashed corned beef and cook for 2–3 minutes until softened and hot. Add 10 halved cherry tomatoes and 2 teaspoons Dijon mustard and stir. Place in a shallow gratin dish. Make up 125 g (4 oz) instant mashed potato according to instructions and spoon on top of the corned beef. Sprinkle with 50 g (2 oz) grated Cheddar cheese. Cook under a preheated hot grill for 2 minutes. Serve with baked beans.

 Corned Beef and Tomato Tarts

Unroll 250 g (8 oz) ready-rolled puff pastry and cut into 4 equal rectangles and place on a baking sheet. Lightly score each rectangle 1 cm (½ inch) in from the edge all the way round to produce an inner rectangle (don't cut all the way through). Bake in a preheated oven, 200°C (400°F), Gas Mark 6, for 10–12 minutes until golden and puffed. Meanwhile, heat 1 tablespoon olive oil in a frying pan and cook 1 small finely chopped onion for 3 minutes,

then roughly mash 350 g (11½ oz) canned corned beef with 1 teaspoon Dijon mustard, add to the pan and cook for 4–5 minutes until the corned beef is softened and hot. Stir in 8 halved cherry tomatoes for the final 2 minutes. Add 2 tablespoons chopped parsley. Once the tart bases are cooked, remove from the oven. Remove the inner rectangle of pastry and set aside. Divide the corned beef mixture between the tarts and top with the inner pastry rectangles as lids.

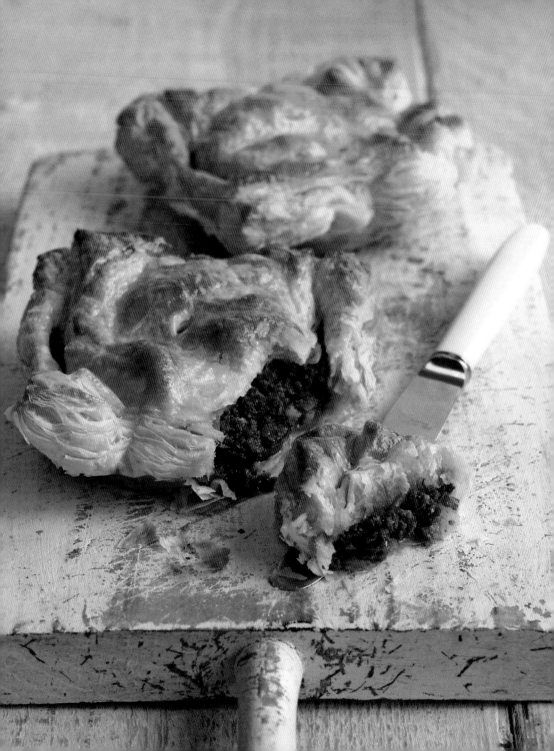

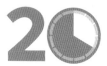

Tuna and Sweetcorn Nuggets

Serves 4

75 g (3 oz) plain flour, plus extra
    for coating
1 large egg
2 tablespoons milk
pinch of chilli powder (optional)
185 g (6½ oz) can tuna, drained
    and flaked
150 g (5 oz) can sweetcorn,
    drained
2 spring onions, chopped
3 tablespoons sunflower oil
salt and pepper
tomato ketchup, to serve

- Place the flour in a bowl and make a well in the centre. Add the egg, milk and chilli powder, if using, and season with salt and pepper. Stir well to make a stiff batter.

- Add the tuna, sweetcorn and spring onions and stir until evenly mixed. Take tablespoons of the mixture, dip them in flour and roughly shape into 16 nuggets.

- Heat the oil in a large frying pan, add the nuggets and fry, in 2 batches, for about 5 minutes, turning occasionally, until golden. Drain on kitchen paper and serve with ketchup.

 Tuna and Sweetcorn Omelette Heat 25 g (1 oz) butter in a nonstick frying pan. Add 2 chopped spring onions and cook for 2 minutes. Beat together 4 eggs, a 185 g (6½ oz) can tuna, drained and flaked, and a 200 g (7 oz) can sweetcorn, drained. Season and pour into the pan. Dot with 4 halved cherry tomatoes and cook until the egg has set underneath, gently pulling the cooked edges towards the centre. When almost set, place the pan under a preheated hot grill (keeping the handle away from the heat) and cook for 2 minutes. Cut into wedges and serve with crusty bread.

 Cheesy Tuna and Sweetcorn Baked Potatoes Scrub 4 small baking potatoes, about 125 g (4 oz) each, and prick all over with a fork. Cook in the microwave on full power for about 15 minutes until soft. Cut in half and scoop the potato into a bowl. Roughly mash the potato with 50 g (2 oz) grated Cheddar cheese and season with salt and pepper. Stir in 2 chopped spring onions, a 185 g (6½ oz) can tuna, drained and flaked, and a 200 g (7 oz) can sweetcorn, drained. Spoon the mixture back into the potato skins, place on a foil-lined grill pan and sprinkle extra cheese on the top. Cook under a preheated medium grill for about 5 minutes until the cheese is melted and bubbling. Serve with peas and chopped tomatoes.

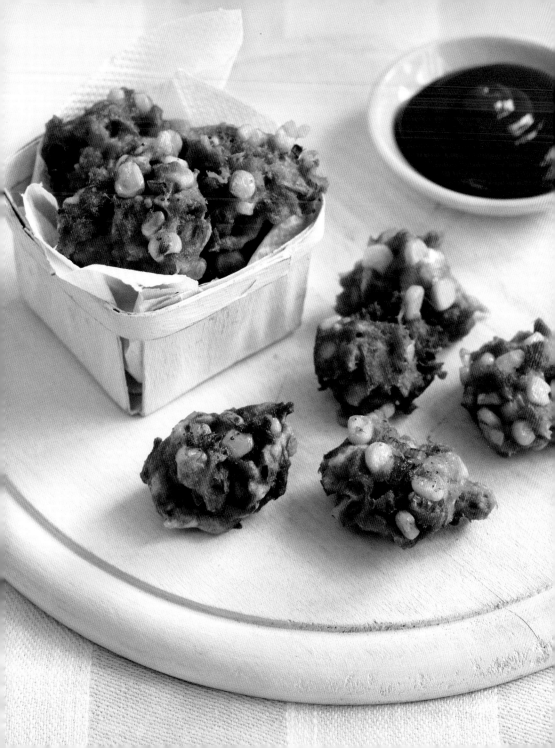

1 Sweet Chilli and Ginger Prawn Vegetable Stir-Fry

Serves 4

500 g (1 lb) ready-cooked rice
1 tablespoon sunflower oil
6 spring onions, each cut into 3
  pieces diagonally, and halved
  lengthways
1 teaspoon ginger purée
125 g (4 oz) sugarsnap peas
125 g (4 oz) frozen soya beans
1 head pak choi, leaves separated,
  and shredded
375 g (12 oz) peeled prawns
2 tablespoons sweet chilli sauce
2 tablespoons soy sauce

- Heat the rice in the microwave according to the packet instructions. Meanwhile, heat the oil in a wok or large frying pan. Add the spring onions, ginger, sugarsnap peas and soya beans and stir-fry over a high heat for 2 minutes.

- Add the pak choi and stir-fry for 1 minute, then add the prawns and cook for a further minute. Mix together the sweet chilli sauce and soy sauce, pour into the wok and heat through. Serve with the rice.

 2 Sweet Chilli and Ginger Prawn Noodles Soak 250 g (8 oz) rice noodles in boiling water for 2 minutes to soften, then drain. Heat 1 tablespoon sunflower oil in a wok or large frying pan, add 6 chopped spring onions, 125 g (4 oz) sugarsnap peas, 1 coarsely grated carrot, 125 g (4 oz) frozen soya beans and 1 head of pak choi, leaves separated, and stir-fry for 2 minutes. Add 375 g (12 oz) cooked peeled prawns and stir-fry for 2 minutes. Add 200 g (7 oz) coconut milk, 2 tablespoons sweet chilli sauce, 2 tablespoons soy sauce and 1 teaspoon ginger purée, bring to the boil and simmer gently for 5 minutes. Add the noodles, stir through and heat for 2 minutes.

 3 Sweet Chilli and Ginger Prawn Skewers with Fried Rice Mix together 2 tablespoons sweet chilli sauce, 2 tablespoons soy sauce, 1 teaspoon ginger purée from a tube or jar and the juice of ½ lime. Add 375 g (12 oz) large peeled prawns and stir to coat in the mixture, then leave to marinate for 10 minutes. Meanwhile, cook 200 g (7 oz) long grain rice in a saucepan of lightly salted boiling water for about 10 minutes until tender, then drain. Heat 1 tablespoon sunflower oil in a wok or large frying pan, add 6 chopped spring onions, 125 g (4 oz) sugarsnap peas, 1 coarsely grated carrot, 125 g (4 oz) frozen soya beans and 1 head of pak choi, leaves separated, and stir-fry over a high heat for 2 minutes until the pak choi has started to wilt. Stir in the drained rice and 2 tablespoons soy sauce and heat through for 2 minutes. Thread the prawns on to skewers and cook under a preheated medium grill for 5 minutes, turning occasionally until pink and hot. Serve with the stir-fried rice.

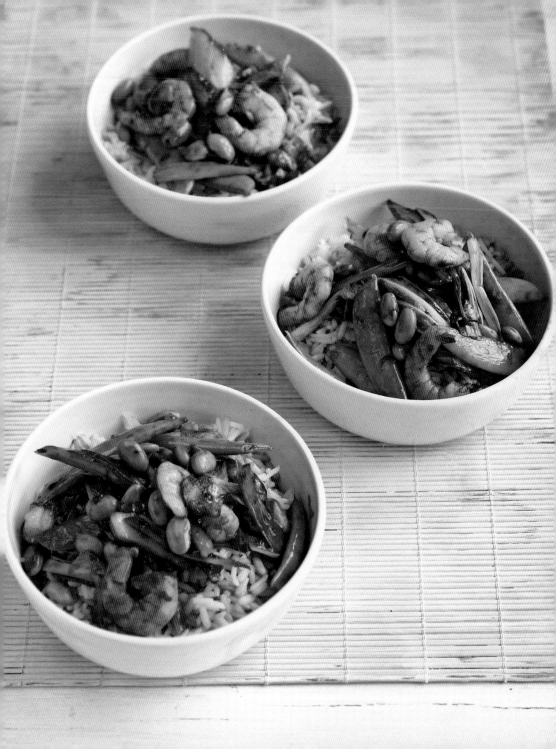

20 Parmesan Chicken Salad

Serves 4

150 g (5 oz) white breadcrumbs
50 g (2 oz) grated Parmesan cheese, grated
2 tablespoons plain flour
1 egg, beaten
4 boneless, skinless chicken breasts, cut in half horizontally
3 tablespoons olive oil
½ cos lettuce, chopped
¼ cucumber, chopped
75 g (3 oz) sugarsnap peas, shredded
8 cherry tomatoes, halved
4 tablespoons ready-made Caesar salad dressing
salt and pepper

- Mix together the breadcrumbs and Parmesan on a plate and season with salt and pepper. Place the flour on another plate and the beaten egg on a third.

- Dip each piece of chicken into the flour, shaking off any excess, then coat in the beaten egg and finally in the breadcrumbs, pressing firmly to coat.

- Heat the oil in a large frying pan and cook the chicken in batches for 3–4 minutes on each side or until golden, crisp and cooked through.

- Meanwhile, mix together the lettuce, cucumber, sugarsnap peas and tomatoes in a salad bowl, then add the Caesar dressing and toss to lightly coat. Serve with the hot chicken.

10 Chicken and Parmesan Ciabattas

Cut 2 boneless, skinless chicken breasts in half horizontally and season. Heat 2 tablespoons olive oil in a frying pan and cook the chicken for about 5 minutes, turning once, until golden and cooked through. Toast 8 slices of ciabatta on both sides. Top 4 slices with shredded crisp lettuce, a drizzle of ready-made Caesar salad dressing and the hot chicken. Add 2 slices of tomato to each and sprinkle with Parmesan cheese shavings. Cover with the remaining bread.

30 Baked Parmesan Chicken with

Roasted Veg Cut 2 parsnips and 2 carrots into quarters lengthways. Place on a baking sheet with 200 g (7 oz) halved new potatoes. Drizzle over 2 tablespoons olive oil and season with salt and pepper. Roast in a preheated oven, 220°C (425°F), Gas Mark 7, for 25 minutes, turning occasionally, until tender. Meanwhile, cut 3 boneless, skinless chicken breasts into chunky strips. Dip the chicken in beaten egg, then coat in a mixture of 4 tablespoons uncooked couscous and 4 tablespoons grated Parmesan cheese. Spread the chicken out in a single layer on a nonstick baking sheet and cook in the oven with the vegetables for 20 minutes. Serve the chicken and roasted vegetables with green beans or broccoli.

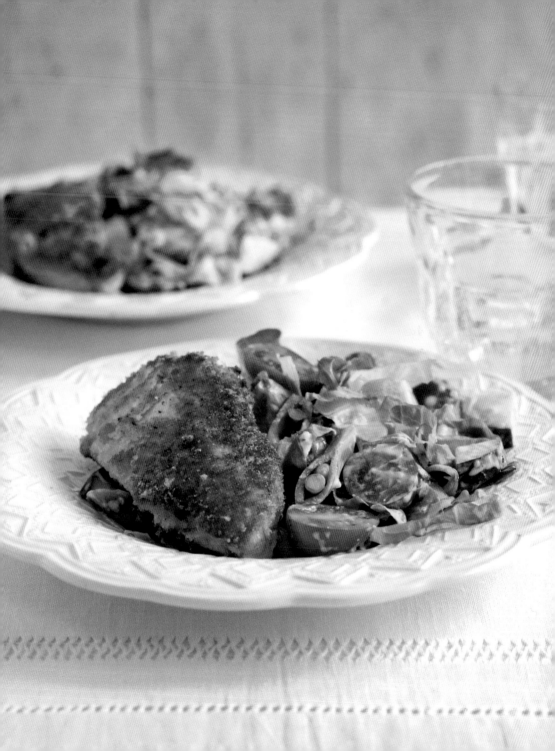

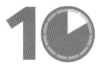

Creamy Tomato Soup with Baked Tortilla Crisps

Serves 4

2 flour tortillas, cut into triangles

1 tablespoon oil

2 x 400 g (13 oz) cans chopped tomatoes

2 tablespoons crème fraîche

300 ml (½ pint) vegetable stock

2 tablespoons tomato purée

2 tablespoons Worcestershire sauce

2 tablespoons thyme

salt and pepper

- Place the tortilla triangles on a baking sheet and roughly brush with the oil. Season and place in a preheated oven, 200°C (400°F), for 8 minutes.

- Meanwhile, place all the remaining ingredients in a saucepan and bring to the boil. Reduce the heat and simmer for 3–4 minutes, then transfer to a food processor and whizz until smooth.

- Serve the soup in mugs with the warm baked tortillas to the side.

---

2 Grilled Creamy Tomato Tortillas

Heat 1 tablespoon oil in a saucepan and cook 1 roughly chopped onion for 3 minutes. Add a 400 g (13 oz) can chopped tomatoes, 2 tablespoons tomato purée, 2 tablespoons Worcestershire sauce and 2 tablespoons thyme and bring to the boil, then remove from the heat. Place 1 flour tortilla on a board and spoon in a quarter of the tomato mixture. Fold the tortilla into 4, enclosing the filling, and place in a shallow gratin dish. Repeat with 3 more. Season 200 ml (7 fl oz) crème fraîche with pepper and place spoonfuls over the tortillas. Scatter with 75 g (3 oz) grated Cheddar cheese and grill for 5–8 minutes.

3 Creamy Tomato Stew with Dumplings

Heat 1 tablespoon olive oil in a large saucepan (with a tight-fitting lid) and cook 1 large chopped onion for 3–4 minutes. Add 500 g (1 lb) whole cherry tomatoes and cook for 2 minutes. Add 2 tablespoons tomato purée, 2 tablespoons Worcestershire sauce, 2 tablespoons thyme and 600 ml (1 pint) vegetable stock and bring to the boil. Reduce the heat, cover and simmer for 5 minutes. Meanwhile, make up a 140 g (4½ oz) packet dumpling mix according to the packet instructions, adding ½ teaspoon dried thyme to the dry mixture. Blend 3 tablespoons cornflour with 4 tablespoons water, add to the tomatoes and stir well to thicken. Add small teaspoons of the dumpling mixture to the pan, cover tightly and simmer for 15 minutes until the dumplings are cooked through. Serve the tomato stew and dumplings with spoonfuls of crème fraîche as a delicious vegetarian supper.

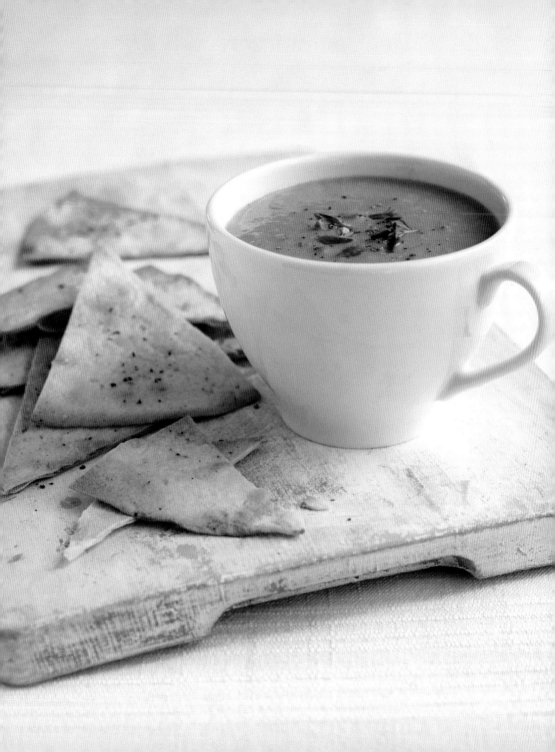

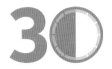 # Mexican Chicken and Avocado Burgers with Salsa

Serves 4

500 g (1 lb) boneless, skinless
   chicken breast, roughly chopped
1 teaspoon dried oregano
1 teaspoon ground cumin
1 teaspoon paprika
½ teaspoon dried chilli flakes
1 tablespoon sunflower oil
4 burger buns
1 avocado, sliced
salt and pepper

For the salsa

2 ripe tomatoes, chopped
½ small red onion, chopped
small bunch of coriander,
   chopped
juice of 1 lime

- Place the chicken in a food processor with the oregano, cumin, paprika and chilli flakes. Season with salt and pepper and whizz until finely chopped. Shape the mixture into 4 burgers and set aside.

- To make the salsa, mix together the tomatoes, red onion, coriander and lime juice and season with salt and pepper.

- Heat the oil in a large frying pan, add the chicken burgers and cook for 5–8 minutes on each side until golden and cooked through.

- Halve and toast the cut sides of the burger buns. Serve the burgers in the buns topped with slices of avocado and a spoonful of salsa.

 ### Chicken and Avocado Quesadillas

Spread 2 soft flour tortillas with 4 tablespoons ready-made tomato salsa. Top with 200 g (7 oz) chopped cooked chicken, 1 sliced avocado and 125 g (4 oz) grated Cheddar cheese. Place another tortilla on the top of each. Heat a large frying pan until hot, then cook the tortilla sandwiches one at a time for about 5 minutes, turning once, until the tortillas are crisp and the cheese has started to melt. Serve cut into wedges with cucumber and carrot sticks.

Avocado and Mozzarella Chicken

Cut 2 boneless, skinless chicken breasts in half horizontally. Season the chicken with a sprinkle of fajita seasoning mix and fry in 2 tablespoons sunflower oil for about 8 minutes, turning once, until golden and cooked through. Top each piece of chicken with 2 slices of tomato, 2–3 slices of avocado and 2 slices of mozzarella cheese. Place the pan under a preheated medium grill (keeping the handle away from the heat) for 3–4 minutes until the cheese melts and starts to brown. Serve with oven chips.

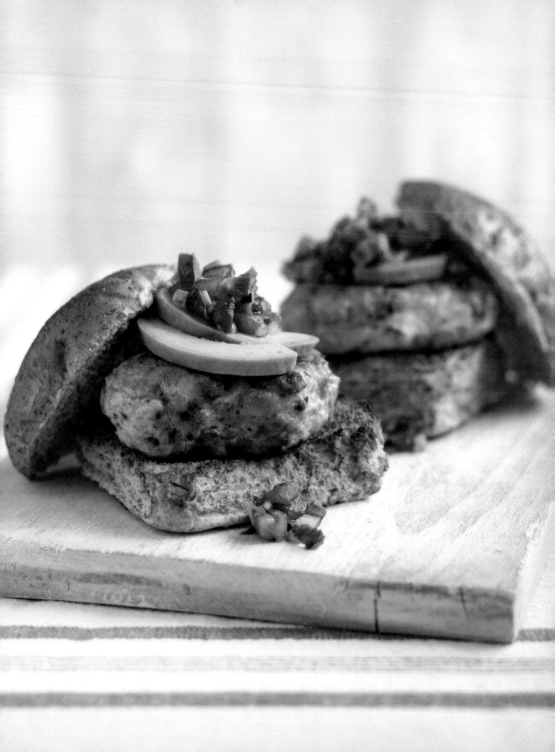

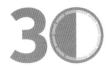 # Easy Ham and Veg Scone Pizzas

Makes 4

175 g (6 oz) plain flour, plus extra
for dusting
200 g (7 oz) wholemeal flour
1 tablespoon demerara sugar
1 teaspoon bicarbonate of soda
250 ml (8 fl oz) buttermilk
2 tablespoons olive oil
1 red pepper, cored, deseeded and
cut into strips
1 large courgette, sliced diagonally
150 ml (¼ pint) ready-made
tomato pizza sauce
handful of spinach leaves
75 g (3 oz) wafer-thin ham
300 g (10 oz) mozzarella cheese,
drained and sliced

- Place the 2 flours in a large bowl with the sugar and bicarbonate of soda and mix well. Add the buttermilk and mix well to form a dough. Turn out on to a floured surface and knead briefly. Divide the dough into 4 pieces, then roll out each piece to about a 15 cm (6 inch) thin round and place on 2 baking sheets.

- Heat the oil in a large frying pan and fry the pepper and courgette over a high heat for 5 minutes.

- Meanwhile, spread each pizza base with 3–4 tablespoons of the tomato sauce to within 2.5 cm (1 inch) of the edge. Top each with spinach, ham, courgette and peppers, then arrange the mozzarella slices over the top.

- Bake at the top of a preheated oven, 220°C (425°F), Gas Mark 7, for 10–12 minutes until golden and the top is melted.

1 Simple Ham and Pepper Melts

Cut 4 ready-made cheese scones in half and place in a shallow gratin dish. Drain a 300 g (10 oz) jar mixed antipasti peppers, then roughly chop, mix with 2 handfuls of spinach leaves and scatter over the scones. Arrange 75 g (3 oz) roughly chopped wafer-thin ham on top, then scatter with 5 tablespoons grated mozzarella cheese. Cook under a preheated hot grill for 4–5 minutes and spoon on to serving plates.

2 Courgette, Ham and Pepper Pizza with Soft Cheese

Place 4 ready-made pizza bases on 2 baking sheets, spread each with 3 tablespoons ready-made tomato pizza sauce and set aside. Heat 2 tablespoons olive oil in a frying pan and cook 1 small cored, deseeded and roughly chopped red pepper, 1 small roughly chopped yellow pepper and 1 thinly sliced courgette over a high heat for 5 minutes until softened and slightly golden in places.

Arrange over the pizza bases with a handful of spinach leaves and 75 g (3 oz) wafer-thin ham, then top each with 2 tablespoons grated mozzarella cheese. Bake in a preheated oven, 220°C (425°F), Gas Mark 7, for 10 minutes until the topping is golden and melted.

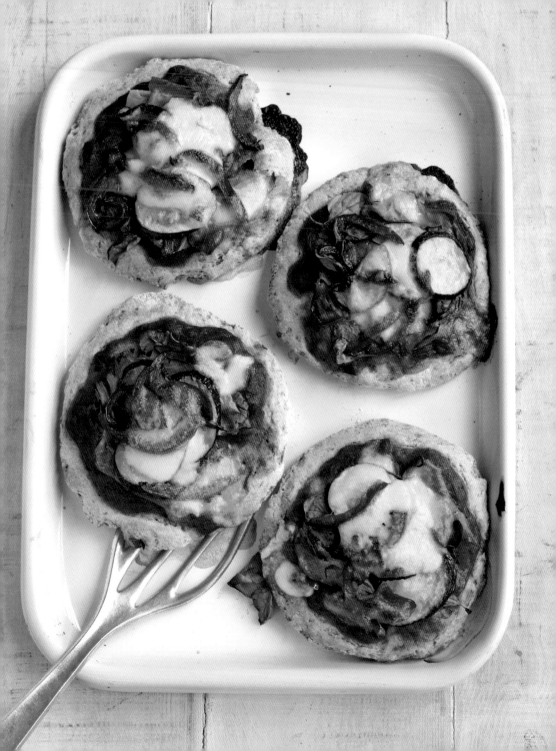

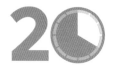

Creamy Chicken, Mushroom and Broccoli Pasta Gratin

Serves 4

250 g (8 oz) pasta shapes
200 g (7 oz) broccoli florets
2 tablespoons olive oil
250 g (8 oz) chicken breasts, cut into thin strips
175 g (6 oz) chestnut mushrooms, thickly sliced or quartered
400 ml (14 fl oz) crème fraîche
1 tablespoon Dijon mustard
4 tablespoons wholemeal breadcrumbs
4 tablespoons grated Parmesan cheese
watercress salad, to serve

- Cook the pasta in a large saucepan of lightly salted boiling water for 5 minutes. Add the broccoli and cook for a further 5 minutes.

- Meanwhile, heat the oil in a large heavy-based frying pan and cook the chicken over a high heat for 5 minutes. Add the mushrooms and cook for a further 3–4 minutes until both are golden and cooked. Add the crème fraîche and Dijon mustard and heat and stir for 1 minute until loosened and mixed together well.

- Drain the pasta and broccoli well, toss into the frying pan and stir. Transfer to a large gratin dish, scatter with the breadcrumbs and Parmesan and cook under a preheated hot grill for 2–3 minutes until golden and bubbling.

- Serve with a simple watercress salad.

 Creamy Chicken and Mushroom Pasta Cook 375 g (12 oz) pasta shapes in a large saucepan of lightly salted boiling water for 3 minutes or according to the packet instructions. Meanwhile, heat 2 tablespoons olive oil in a frying pan and cook 250 g (8 oz) thinly sliced chicken breast and 175 g (6 oz) quartered chestnut mushrooms over a high heat for 8 minutes until golden and cooked through. Add 400 ml (14 fl oz) crème fraîche and 1 tablespoon Dijon mustard and heat for 1 minute. Drain the pasta, add it to the pan and toss before serving.

 Béchamel Chicken, Mushroom and Broccoli Pasta Gratin Cook 250 g (8 oz) pasta shapes in a large saucepan of lightly salted boiling water for 8–10 minutes, adding 250 g (8 oz) broccoli florets for the final 5 minutes. Drain. In a separate frying pan, heat 2 tablespoons olive oil and cook 250 g (8 oz) thinly sliced chicken breast over a high heat for 8–10 minutes until golden and cooked through. Meanwhile, heat 50 g (2 oz) butter in a large heavy-based frying pan and cook 200 g (7 oz) roughly chopped mushrooms over a high heat for 5 minutes until golden. Add 2 tablespoons plain flour and stir well to mix, then return to the heat for 30 seconds, stirring. Remove from the heat and add 300 ml (½ pint) milk, a little at a time, stirring well between each addition until smooth. Return to the heat and bring to the boil, stirring well until boiled and thickened. Add 400 ml (14 fl oz) crème fraîche, then mix with the pasta, broccoli and chicken. Pile into a large gratin dish and top with 4 tablespoons wholemeal breadcrumbs and 4 tablespoons grated Parmesan cheese mixed together. Cook under a preheated grill for 3–4 minutes until golden and bubbling.

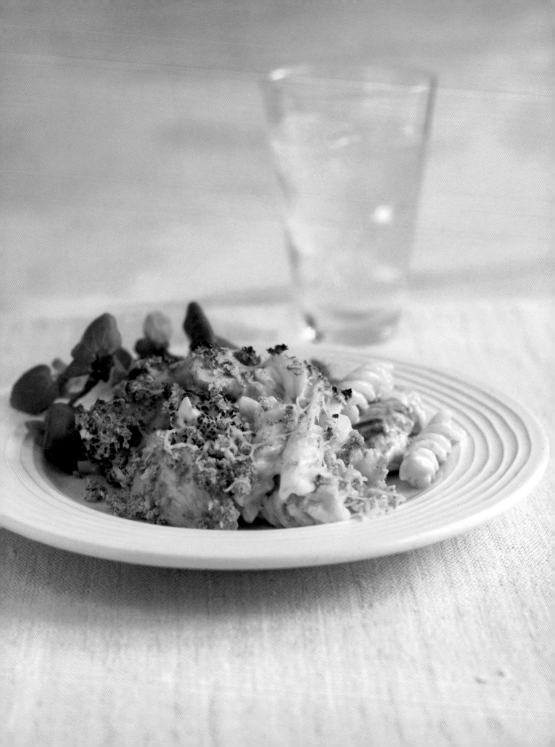

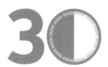

Shepherd's Pie (with Hidden Veg!)

Serves 4

500 g (1 lb) swede, peeled and
cut into rough chunks

3 carrots, peeled and cut into
chunks, plus 1 large carrot,
peeled and grated

375 g (12 oz) good-quality
minced lamb

1 courgette, grated

1 beef stock cube, crumbled

400 g (13 oz) can chopped
tomatoes

4 tablespoons Worcestershire
sauce

3 tablespoons tomato purée

25 g (1 oz) butter

25 g (1 oz) Parmesan cheese,
grated

green vegetables, to serve

- Cook the swede and carrot chunks in a large saucepan of lightly salted boiling water for 15–20 minutes until tender.

- Meanwhile, heat a large frying pan for 1 minute. Add the mince and dry-fry over a high heat for 5 minutes until browned, stirring frequently. Add the grated carrot and courgette and cook for 3 minutes, then add the stock cube, tomatoes, Worcestershire sauce and tomato purée. Stir well, then bring to the boil. Reduce the heat, cover and simmer for 10 minutes.

- Drain the swede and carrots, add the butter and mash well using a potato masher or electric blender until thick and almost smooth.

- Spoon the meat into a shallow gratin dish and spoon the swede mash over the top. Scatter over the Parmesan and cook under a preheated grill for 3–4 minutes until golden. Serve hot with green vegetables.

 Minute Steaks with Vegetable Sauce
Season 4 x 75 g (3 oz) minute steaks with a little pepper. Heat 2 tablespoons olive oil in a large frying pan and cook 1 small roughly chopped courgette and 1 small peeled and roughly chopped carrot for 5 minutes. Meanwhile, cook the steaks under a hot grill on each side for 2–3 minutes. Add 400 g (13 oz) canned chopped tomatoes and 1 tablespoon tomato purée to the vegetables and stir and cook for 2 minutes. Serve the steaks with the sauce spooned over.

 Hidden-Vegetable Mince with Mashed Swede Cook 500 g (1 lb) roughly chopped swede in a saucepan of lightly salted boiling water for 15 minutes until tender. Heat a large heavy-based frying pan for 1 minute. Add 500 g (1 lb) good-quality minced beef and cook over a high heat for 5 minutes until browned. Add 1 trimmed and grated courgette and 1 grated carrot and cook for a further 2 minutes. Add 1 tablespoon tomato purée and 2 tablespoons Worcestershire sauce and cook, stirring, for 2 minutes. Add 1 beef stock cube and 300 ml (½ pint) water, bring to the boil and cook for 5 minutes. Blend 1 tablespoon cornflour with 2 tablespoons water and add to the pan, cooking for 2 minutes and stirring to make a gravy. Drain the swede and mash with 25 g (1 oz) butter. Serve spooned on to warmed serving plates with a ladleful of mince with gravy.

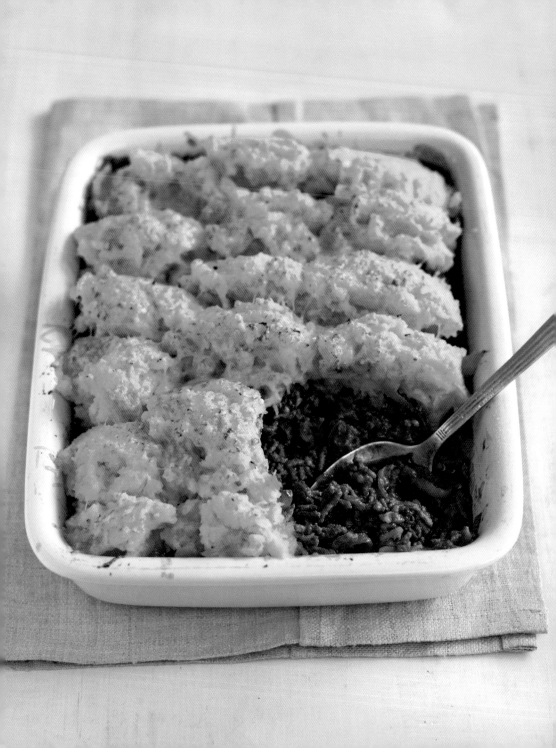

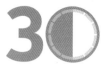

Pork Escalopes with Tomato Pasta

Serves 4

2 pork escalopes, about 175 g
(6 oz) each, halved
2 eggs, beaten
125 g (4 oz) breadcrumbs
375 g (12 oz) spaghetti
1 small onion, chopped
1 garlic clove, crushed
5 ripe tomatoes, chopped
½ teaspoon caster sugar
small handful of basil leaves, torn
3 tablespoons sunflower oil
salt and pepper
grated cheese, to serve

- Place the escalope halves between sheets of clingfilm and bash with a rolling pin until 5–8 mm (⅛–⅓ inch) thick. Place the beaten eggs on one plate and the breadcrumbs on another and season well. Dip the pork in the egg to coat, then the breadcrumbs, pressing firmly to coat.

- Cook the spaghetti in a saucepan of lightly salted boiling water for about 10 minutes until just tender.

- Heat 1 tablespoon of the oil in a frying pan, add the onion and garlic and cook for 5 minutes until softened. Add the tomatoes and sugar and season with salt and pepper. Cook for about 5 minutes until the tomatoes are soft and pulpy. Stir in the basil.

- Meanwhile heat the remaining oil in a large frying pan, add the pork escalopes and fry, in batches, 2 at a time for 3 minutes on each side until golden, crisp and cooked through.

- Drain the spaghetti, mix with the tomato sauce, sprinkle with grated cheese and serve with the pork escalopes.

 Pork and Cherry Tomato Stir-Fry
Cut 4 boneless pork steaks, about 125 g (4 oz) each, into strips and stir-fry in 2 tablespoons sunflower oil over a high heat for 2 minutes. Add 8 cherry tomatoes and stir-fry for 1 minute, then stir in 350 g (11½ oz) ready-made tomato and herb pasta sauce and 200 g (7 oz) ready-cooked rice. Stir well and heat through until piping hot. Serve with crusty bread.

 Pan-Fried Pork with Creamy Tomato Sauce Thickly slice 500 g (1 lb) pork tenderloin fillet and fry in 2 tablespoons olive oil for about 5 minutes, turning once, until browned and cooked through. Remove from the pan and set aside. Add 1 crushed garlic clove, 300 ml (½ pint) passata and 125 g (4 oz) mascarpone cheese to the pan. Bring to the boil, stirring, then season with salt and pepper and return the pork to the pan. Heat through for a few minutes, then serve with peas and oven chips or potato wedges.

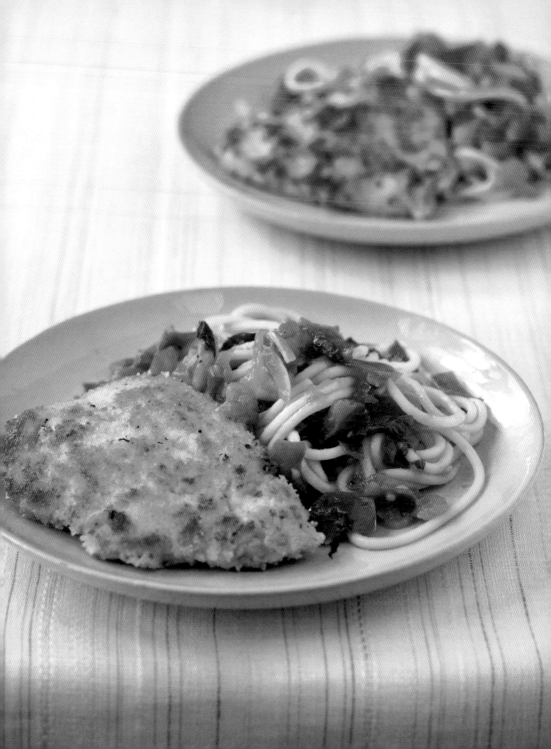

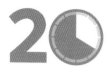

Sweetcorn Fritters with Tomato Salsa

Makes 16

125 g (4 oz) plain flour

1 egg

150 ml (¼ pint) milk

400 g (13 oz) canned sweetcorn, drained

4 tablespoons sunflower oil

salt and pepper

ready-made guacamole, to serve

For the salsa

3 ripe tomatoes, chopped

2 spring onions, chopped

pinch of caster sugar

2 tablespoons ready-made French dressing

- Place the flour in a bowl, make a well in the centre and break in the egg. Gradually add the milk, mixing with a hand whisk to make a smooth thick batter. Season with salt and pepper and stir in the sweetcorn.

- Heat the oil in a large frying pan, add spoonfuls of the batter and fry, in batches, for about 5 minutes, turning once, until golden and crisp. Drain on kitchen paper.

- To make the salsa, place the tomatoes in a bowl and crush lightly with a fork. Add the spring onions, sugar and French dressing, season with salt and pepper and mix well.

- Serve the fritters with the tomato salsa and guacamole.

 Sweetcorn and Mixed Bean Tacos

Mix together a 200 g (7 oz) can sweetcorn, drained, and a 300 g (10 oz) can spicy mixed beans, rinsed and drained, in a bowl. Spoon into 4 taco shells with ¼ shredded iceberg lettuce, 2 grated carrots and a sprinkle of grated cheese. Serve with tomato salsa and soured cream.

 Sweetcorn, Bacon and Cheese Tarts

Cook 4 bacon rashers under a preheated hot grill until crisp, then chop and set aside. Unroll 1 sheet of ready-rolled puff pastry, cut into 4 equal squares and place on a baking sheet lined with baking paper. Mix together 350 g (11½ oz) ready-made cheese sauce, a 200 g (7 oz) can sweetcorn, drained, and the chopped cooked bacon. Spoon the mixture on to the pastry squares and spread evenly, leaving a 1 cm (½ inch) border at the edge. Sprinkle with 50 g (2 oz) grated Cheddar cheese and bake in a preheated oven, 200°C (400°F), Gas Mark 6, for 15–20 minutes until well risen and golden. Serve warm with salad.

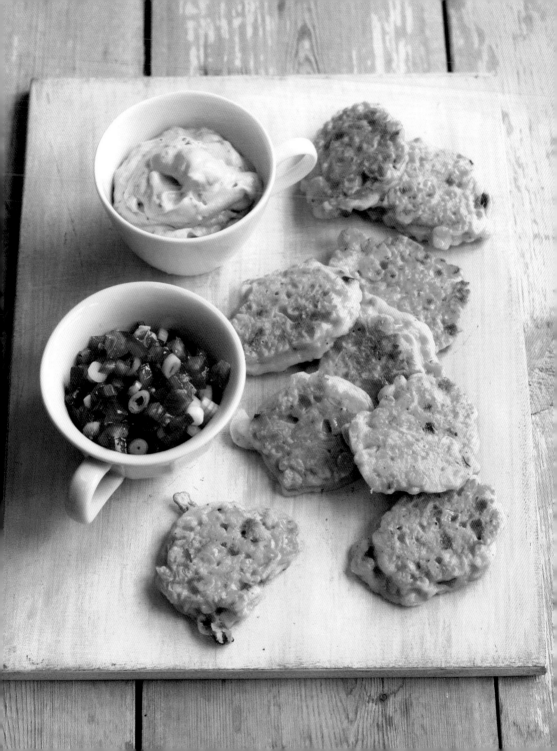

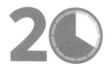

Singapore Noodles

Serves 4

2 tablespoons dark soy sauce

1 teaspoon light muscovado sugar

4 tablespoons water

250 g (8 oz) thin rice noodles

3 tablespoons sunflower oil

2 eggs, lightly beaten

1 onion, finely sliced

1 green pepper, cored, deseeded and cut into strips

200 g (7 oz) cooked, peeled prawns, defrosted if frozen

2.5 cm (1 inch) piece of fresh root ginger, peeled and grated

2 teaspoons medium curry powder

½ small cabbage, finely shredded

salt and pepper

- In a small bowl, mix together the soy sauce, sugar and measurement water and set aside.

- Soak the noodles in boiling water from the kettle for 2 minutes to soften, then drain well.

- Heat 1 tablespoon of the oil in a wok or large frying pan. Add the beaten eggs, season with salt and pepper and cook, stirring, for 1–2 minutes until a flat omelette is formed. Remove from the pan, cut into strips and set aside.

- Heat the remaining oil in the pan, add the onion and green pepper and stir-fry for 2 minutes to soften. Add the prawns, ginger, curry powder and cabbage and cook for a further 2 minutes.

- Stir in the soy sauce mixture and noodles and heat through. Add the scrambled egg and lightly stir through. Serve in bowls and top with the egg strips.

 Spicy Prawn and Pea Noodles

Soak 85 g (3 oz) instant curry-flavoured noodles in boiling water from the kettle according to the the packet instructions. Meanwhile, fry 175 g (6 oz) button mushrooms, halved if large, 100 g (3½ oz) frozen peas and 200 g (7 oz) peeled prawns, defrosted if frozen, until the mushrooms are browned and the peas are cooked (about 3 minutes). Stir into the noodles and serve with a dash of soy sauce.

 Singapore Noodle Stir-Fry

Place 200 g (7 oz) cooked peeled prawns, defrosted if frozen, in a shallow dish. Pour over a mixture of 2 tablespoons dark soy sauce, 1 teaspoon light muscovado sugar, 2.5 cm (1 inch) piece of fresh root ginger, peeled and grated, 2 teaspoons medium curry powder and 4 tablespoons water. Mix well and set aside for 15 minutes. Meanwhile, soak 250 g (8 oz) thin rice noodles in boiling water from the kettle for 2 minutes to soften, then drain. Heat 2 tablespoons sunflower oil in a wok or large frying pan. Add 1 sliced onion and 1 green pepper, cored, deseeded and cut into strips, and stir-fry for 5 minutes until softened. Remove the prawns from the marinade (reserving the marinade), add to the pan and stir-fry for 2 minutes, then stir in the reserved marinade and bring to the boil. Add the noodles, toss lightly to mix and heat through.

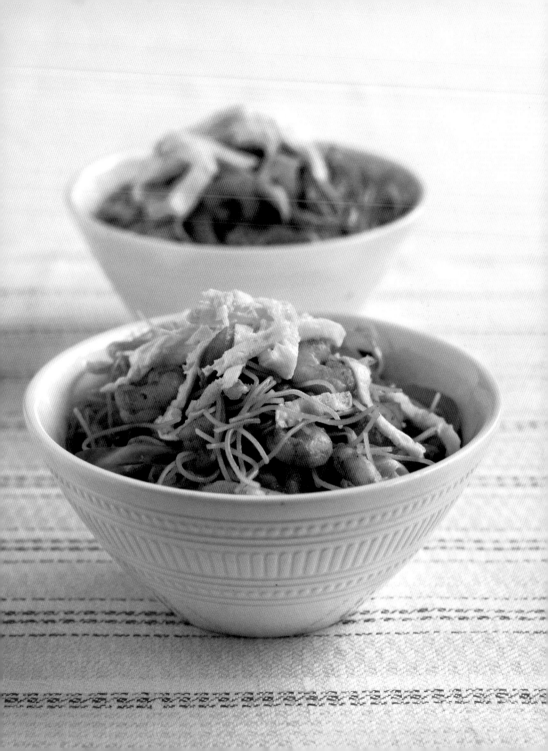

30 Fish Fingers with Sweet Potato Chips

Serves 4

4 sweet potatoes, cut into slim
wedges

2 tablespoons olive oil

500 g (1 lb) cod loin, cut into
2.5 cm (1 inch) strips

125 g (4 oz) plain flour

175 g (6 oz) wholemeal
breadcrumbs

3 tablespoons chopped parsley,
plus extra to garnish (optional)

2 eggs, beaten

salt and pepper

tartare sauce, to serve

- Place the sweet potato wedges in a bowl with the oil and toss well to coat, then season with a little salt and pepper. Transfer to a baking sheet and cook in a preheated oven, 200°C (400°F), Gas Mark 6, for 20 minutes.

- Meanwhile, toss the fish strips in the flour. Place the breadcrumbs in a bowl and toss well. Working quickly, take a floured fish strip and dip in the egg, then in the herby breadcrumbs, and place on a baking sheet. Continue until all are used, then bake in the oven for 15 minutes until the breadcrumbs are golden and the fish is opaque and cooked through.

- Serve with the sweet potato wedges and tartare sauce, with parsley.

 Fish Fingers with Sweet Potato Mash

Bring a pan of lightly salted water to the boil. Meanwhile, peel 3 sweet potatoes and roughly chop into small pieces. Add to the pan and cook for 8 minutes. Meanwhile, cook 8 frozen fish fingers under a preheated hot grill for 6–7 minutes, turning once, until golden and cooked through. Drain the potatoes and add 25 g (1 oz) butter. Mash with a potato masher until rough-textured. Stir in 2 tablespoons chopped parsley and season with pepper. Spoon on to warmed serving plates and serve with the fish fingers.

 Roasted Sweet Potato and Cod with a Crunchy Topping

Cut 2 sweet potatoes into small cubes. Place in a roasting tin, drizzle with 2 tablespoons olive oil and toss well to coat. Roast in the top of a preheated oven, 220°C (425°F), Gas Mark 7, for 15–18 minutes. Meanwhile, place 4 small cod loins, about 125 g (4 oz) each, on a separate roasting tray and season generously with pepper. Mix 2 tablespoons wholemeal breadcrumbs with 1 tablespoon chopped parsley and scatter over the fish. Roast in the oven with the potatoes for 10–12 minutes until the fish is opaque and cooked through and the breadcrumbs have turned golden and crunchy in places. Serve with the sweet potato cubes with spoonfuls of tartare sauce or mayonnaise, if liked.

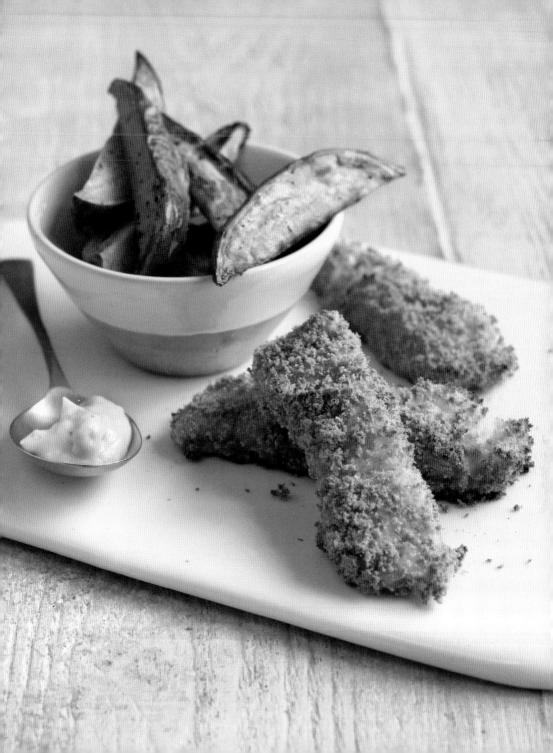

30 Sausage, Courgette and Tomato Risotto

Serves 4

4 thick pork sausages
2 tablespoon olive oil
1 onion, chopped
1 courgette, chopped
175 g (6 oz) Arborio risotto rice
400 g (13 oz) can chopped
  tomatoes
750 ml (1¼ pints) hot chicken
  stock
50 g (2 oz) Parmesan cheese,
  grated, plus extra to serve
salt and pepper
garlic bread, to serve

- Cook the sausages under a preheated grill for 10 minutes, turning occasionally, until browned and cooked through.

- Meanwhile, heat the oil in a large, deep frying pan or shallow saucepan. Add the onion and courgette and fry for 5 minutes to soften. Add the rice and stir well. Stir in the tomatoes and half the stock. Bring to the boil, stirring occasionally, and simmer until almost all the stock has been absorbed. Add the remaining stock and simmer, stirring occasionally, until the rice is tender and the stock has been absorbed.

- Slice the cooked sausages and stir into the risotto with the Parmesan. Season with salt and pepper and serve with extra Parmesan and garlic bread.

 Sausage and Courgette Ciabatta Pizzas Cut a ciabatta loaf in half horizontally, place on a baking sheet and spread the cut sides with 3 tablespoons ready-made pizza sauce. Chop 12 cooked cocktail sausages and scatter over the tops with ½ thinly sliced courgette. Sprinkle over 125 g (4 oz) ready-grated pizza cheese and bake in a preheated oven, 220°C (425°F), Gas Mark 7, for 8 minutes until the cheese has melted and bread is crisp.

Sausage, Courgette and Tomato Kebabs Cut 8 chipolatas into thirds and thread on to skewers alternately with 8 cherry tomatoes and 1 thickly sliced courgette. Brush with some ready-made barbecue sauce and cook under a preheated grill for about 10 minutes, turning occasionally, until the sausages are cooked and the courgette is tender. Serve with rice, sweetcorn and extra barbecue sauce.

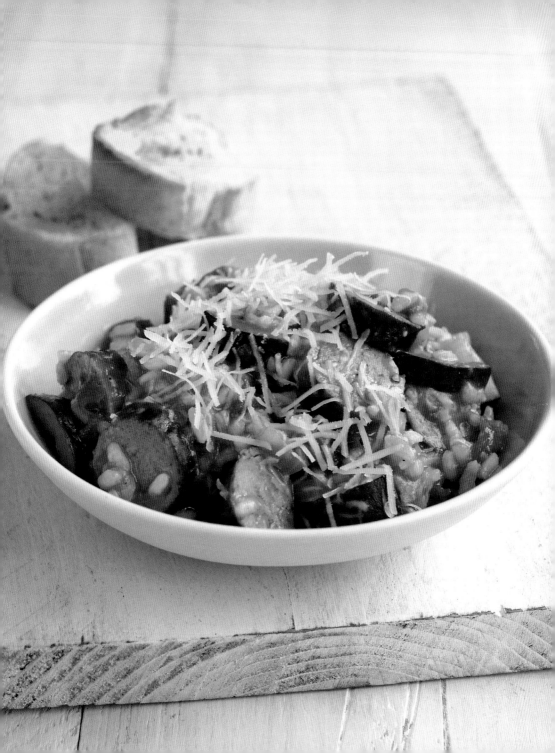

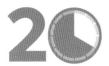 # Bubble and Squeak Patties

Makes 8

2 tablespoons olive oil

1 red onion, finely sliced

200 g (7 oz) savoy cabbage, chunky stems removed and shredded

400 g (13 oz) ready-made mashed potato

1 tablespoon Dijon mustard

50 g (2 oz) Gruyère cheese, finely grated

1 egg yolk

75 g (3 oz) seasoned flour

4 tablespoons vegetable oil

rich tomato sauce, to serve

- Heat the olive oil in a large heavy-based frying pan and cook the onion over a medium heat for 3 minutes until beginning to soften. Add the cabbage and cook, stirring, for a further 3–4 minutes until softened and beginning to turn golden.

- Place the mashed potato in a large mixing bowl, add the Dijon mustard and Gruyère and mix well, then add the egg yolk and mix again. Add the warm cabbage and onion mixture and stir again, then divide the mix into 8 pieces. Shape into patties using floured hands, then dip each one in a little seasoned flour and set aside.

- Heat the vegetable oil in a large heavy-based frying pan and cook the patties over a medium heat for 2–3 minutes on each side until golden. Serve hot with rich tomato sauce.

10 Potato and Cabbage Soup

Place 250 g (8 oz) savoy cabbage in a pan with 600 ml (1 pint) chicken or vegetable stock and bring to the boil. Add 250 g (8 oz) chilled ready-made mashed potato and 1 tablespoon Dijon mustard and cook, stirring, for a further 5 minutes. Transfer the mixture to a food processor and whizz until smooth. Serve in warmed serving bowls with ready-made croutons and grated cheese scattered over.

30 Cheesy Bubble and Squeak

Heat 4 tablespoons olive oil and 15 g (½ oz) butter in a large heavy-based frying pan and cook 1 sliced red onion for 5 minutes until softened and golden. Add 500 g (1 lb) chilled ready-made mashed potato and cook over a high heat for 10 minutes, stirring occasionally, until golden and crisp in places (the secret of a good bubble and squeak is to get the potato crispy, and this takes time to perfect without burning). Add 250 g (8 oz) shredded savoy cabbage and cook for a further 6–7 minutes until softened, stirring occasionally. Scatter over 125 g (4 oz) grated Cheddar cheese. Place the pan under a preheated hot grill, keeping the handle away from the heat, and cook for 5 minutes until golden. Serve in wedges.

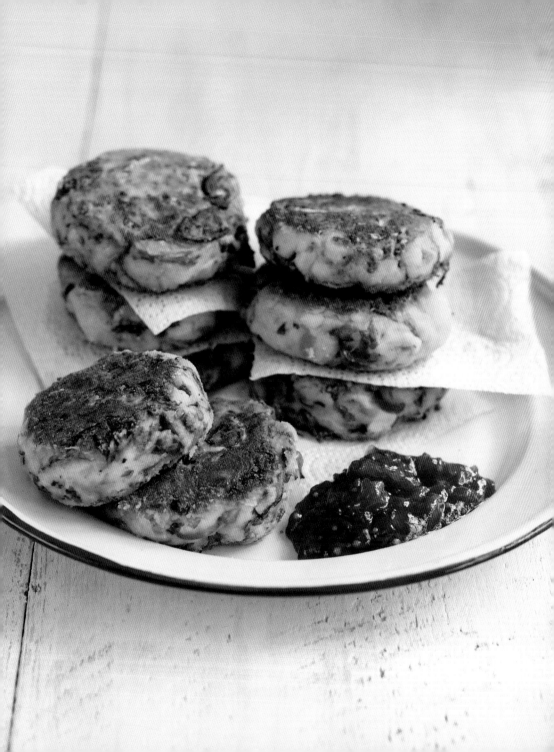

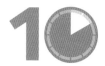

Creamy Garlic Mushroom Bagels

Serves 2

1 tablespoon olive oil

150 g (5 oz) button mushrooms, halved if large

75 g (3 oz) garlic and herb soft cheese

2–3 tablespoons milk

2 bagels

50 g (2 oz) Cheddar cheese, grated, to serve

- Heat the oil in a frying pan. Add the mushrooms and cook over a high heat for 3–4 minutes until golden and tender. Reduce the heat and stir in the soft cheese and milk to make a creamy sauce, adding a little more milk if necessary.

- Meanwhile, halve and toast the bagels under a preheated grill. Spoon the creamy mushrooms on top and sprinkle with the Cheddar cheese to serve.

 Creamy Mushroom Soup with Garlic Bagel Toasts Fry 1 small chopped onion and 250 g (8 oz) chopped mushrooms in 25 g (1 oz) butter for 5 minutes until the onion has softened. Pour in 300 ml (½ pint) vegetable stock, season with salt and pepper and simmer for 5 minutes. Blend with a hand-held blender until almost smooth, stir in 100 ml (3½ fl oz) crème fraîche and reheat. Spread halved bagels with ready-made garlic butter and grill until golden and crisp. Serve the soup with an extra spoonful of crème fraîche and the toasted garlic bagels.

 Baked Garlicky Mozzarella Mushrooms Fry 1 small onion and 3 chopped bacon rashers in 1 tablespoon olive oil for 5 minutes until the onion softens and the bacon is crisp. Add 1 crushed garlic clove and 2 slices of bread, cut into small cubes, and fry for 2 minutes, then remove from the heat and stir in 2 tablespoons chopped parsley. Place 200 g (7 oz) open-cup mushrooms in a baking dish. Scatter the onion mixture over the top, sprinkle with 150 g (5 oz) chopped mozzarella cheese and drizzle with olive oil. Bake in a preheated oven, 200°C (400°F), Gas Mark 6, for 20 minutes until the cheese is melted and golden and the mushrooms are cooked. Serve with salad.

KID-KIDS-MUM

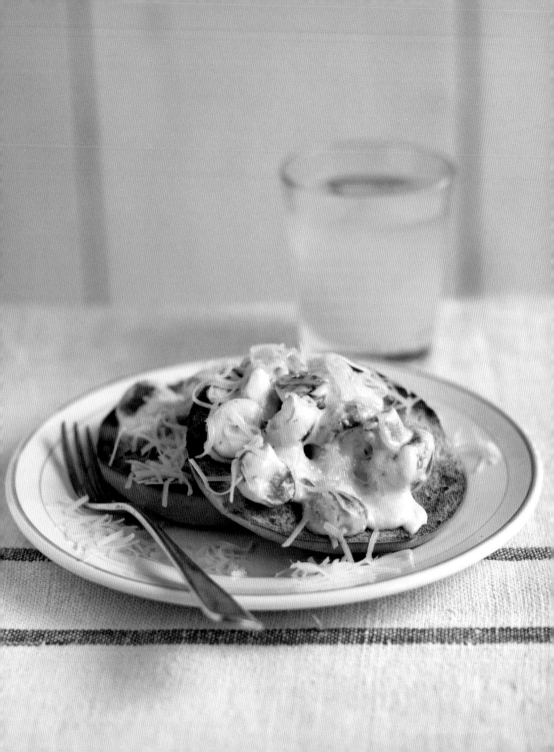

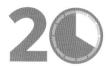 # Hidden Vegetable Pasta

Serves 4

1 tablespoon olive oil

1 onion, chopped

2 carrots, chopped

½ small butternut squash, chopped

1 leek, rinsed, trimmed and chopped

1 courgette, chopped

150 g (5 oz) mushrooms, chopped

500 g (1 lb) passata with garlic and herbs

150 ml (¼ pint) vegetable stock

300 g (10 oz) linguine or tagliatelle

salt and pepper

grated cheese, to serve

- Heat the oil in a large pan. Add the onion, carrots, butternut squash, leek, courgette and mushrooms and cook over a high heat for 5 minutes to soften.

- Add the passata and stock, bring to the boil, then reduce the heat, cover and simmer for 10 minutes. Meanwhile, cook the linguine or tagliatelle in a large saucepan of lightly salted boiling water for 8–10 minutes until tender, then drain and return to the pan.

- Using a hand-held blender or food processor, blend the sauce until smooth, adding a little water if necessary. Season with salt and pepper, then toss with the linguine or tagliatelle. Serve with plenty of grated cheese.

 ### Quick Vegetable Tortelloni Grill

Cook 350 g (11½ oz) spinach and ricotta tortelloni in a saucepan of lightly salted boiling water for 3–4 minutes, then drain. Meanwhile, heat 350 g (11½ oz) ready-made tomato pasta sauce in a saucepan. Add ½ coarsely grated courgette, 1 peeled and grated carrot and 50 g (2 oz) chopped mushrooms and cook for 5 minutes to soften the vegetables. Mix together the tortelloni and sauce, tip into a heatproof dish and top with 150 g (5 oz) sliced mozzarella cheese. Place under a preheated hot grill for 2–3 minutes until the cheese is bubbling.

 ### Hidden Vegetable Pizzas

Heat 1 tablespoon olive oil in a large saucepan, add 1 small chopped onion, 1 peeled and chopped carrot, ¼ peeled and chopped butternut squash, 1 chopped courgette and 50 g (2 oz) chopped mushrooms. Cook, stirring, for 5 minutes to soften, then add a 400 g (13 oz) can chopped tomatoes with garlic and herbs. Bring to the boil, cover and simmer for 10 minutes. Blend until smooth with a hand-held blender or food processor and season with salt and pepper. Spread the sauce on to 4 ready-made pizza bases, top with 150 g (5 oz) sliced mozzarella cheese and bake in a preheated oven, 220 °C (425 °F), Gas Mark 7, for 10 minutes until the cheese has melted and is starting to brown and the bases are crisp. Serve with salad.

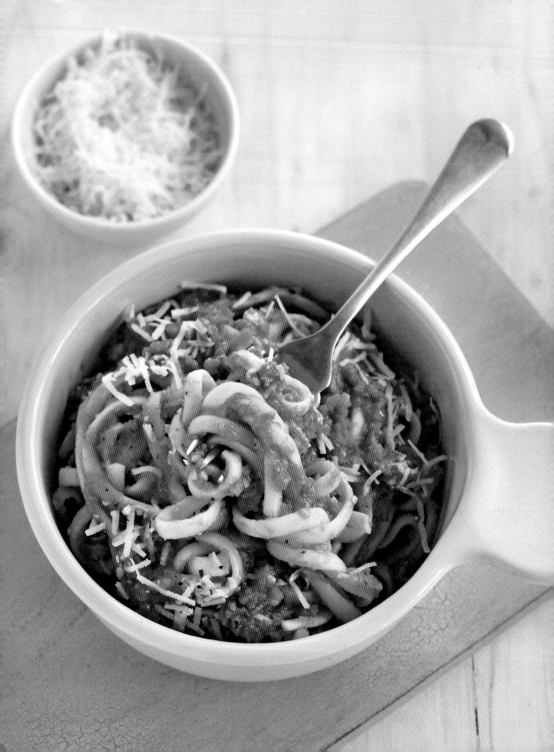

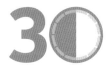

Chicken Nuggets with Sunblush Tomato Sauce

Serves 4

5 tablespoons wholemeal flour
½ teaspoon ground cumin
½ teaspoon ground coriander
½ teaspoon paprika
2 eggs, beaten
2 tablespoons olive oil
450 g (14 ½ oz) chicken breasts
 cut into 3.5 cm (1½ in) chunks
pepper

For the sauce

75 g (3 oz) sunblush tomatoes,
 drained
75 g (3 oz) tomatoes, halved and
 deseeded
2 tablespoons mayonnaise

- Mix together the flour, cumin, coriander and paprika and season with pepper. Divide between 2 plates. Put the beaten egg on a separate plate.

- Pour the oil on to a large baking sheet and heat in a preheated oven, 200°C (400°F), Gas Mark 6, for 5 minutes.

- Meanwhile, one piece at a time, toss the chicken in the first plate of flour, then coat in the egg and then in the second plate of flour. Remove the baking sheet from the oven and toss the nuggets in the oil. Return to the oven and roast for 20 minutes until golden and crisp.

- Meanwhile, to make the sunblush tomato sauce, place both kinds of tomato in a food processor with the mayonnaise and blend until smooth. Remove the nuggets from the oven, drain on kitchen paper and serve with the tomato sauce.

 Spiced Chicken and Sunblush Tomato Pittas Cut 300 g (10 oz) boneless, skinless chicken breasts into thin strips and toss with ½ teaspoon each ground cumin, ground coriander and paprika. Heat 1 tablespoon olive oil in a frying pan and fry the chicken for 7–8 minutes until golden and cooked through, adding 6 roughly chopped sunblush tomatoes for the final minute. Meanwhile, take 4 small pitta breads and lightly toast. Cut open using a serrated knife and fill with salad and the hot chicken and tomato mixture. Serve warm.

 Sunblush Tomato and Spiced Chicken Skewers Cut 3 x 150 g (5 oz) chicken breasts into 2.5 cm (1 inch) chunks, then place in a bowl and toss with ½ teaspoon ground cumin, ½ teaspoon ground coriander and ½ teaspoon paprika. Thread on to 8 wooden or metal skewers, adding 2 sunblush tomatoes and 1 cherry tomato to each skewer. Cook under a preheated medium grill for 8–10 minutes, turning once, until the chicken is cooked and the tomatoes soft. Serve sprinkled with chopped parsley and tomato ketchup.

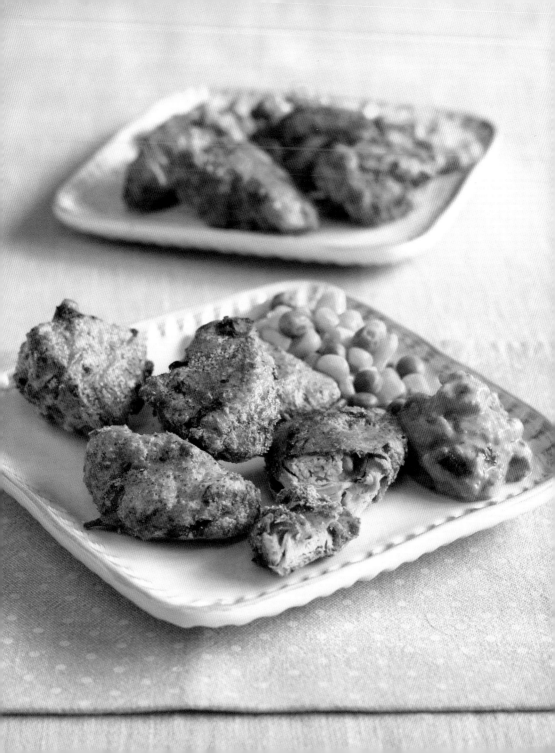

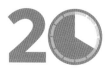 # Bacon, Pea and Potato Frittata

Serves 4

2 tablespoons olive oil

250 g (8 oz) potatoes, cut into small cubes

6 back bacon rashers, roughly snipped

125 g (4 oz) frozen peas

6 tablespoons cold water

6 eggs

1 teaspoon Dijon mustard

pepper

crusty bread, to serve

- Heat the oil in a medium heavy-based frying pan and cook the potatoes over a high heat for 3–4 minutes until golden in places. Add the bacon and cook for a further 5 minutes until golden, stirring occasionally. Add the peas and the measurement water and bring to the boil. Cover with a baking sheet and cook for a further 2–3 minutes.

- Meanwhile, beat the eggs with the mustard and season generously with pepper.

- Remove the baking sheet from the top of the pan, pour in the eggs and mix well to evenly distribute the filling and make sure any surplus water mixes with the eggs. Cook for 2–3 minutes until the base is set, then place the pan under a preheated grill (keeping the handle away from the heat) and cook for a further 2 minutes until the top is golden and set.

- Serve in wedges with crusty bread.

 ### Bacon and Pea Omelette

Heat 1 tablespoon olive oil in a medium heavy-based frying pan and cook 4 roughly chopped bacon rashers over a high heat for 3 minutes until crisp. Add 75 g (3 oz) frozen peas and cook for a further 1 minute. Meanwhile, beat 4 eggs in a small jug, season with pepper and pour into the pan. Gently cook for 2–3 minutes until the base is set, then place the pan under a preheated grill (keeping the handle away from the heat) and cook for 1 minute until the top is set and serve.

 ### Baked Bacon, Pea and Pepper Tortilla

Heat 2 tablespoons olive oil in a frying pan and cook 6 roughly snipped bacon rashers with 1 chopped onion and 1 cored, deseeded and chopped red pepper for 5 minutes. Add 3 roughly chopped tomatoes and 125 g (4 oz) frozen peas and stir and cook for 1 minute, then transfer into a mixing bowl. Beat 8 eggs in a separate jug, season well with pepper, pour into the vegetables and mix well. Lightly grease a 18 x 28 cm (7 x 11 inch) roasting tin with oil, then pour in the egg and vegetable mixture. Bake in a preheated oven, 200°C (400°F), Gas Mark 6, for 20 minutes until golden and puffed. Cut into squares to serve.

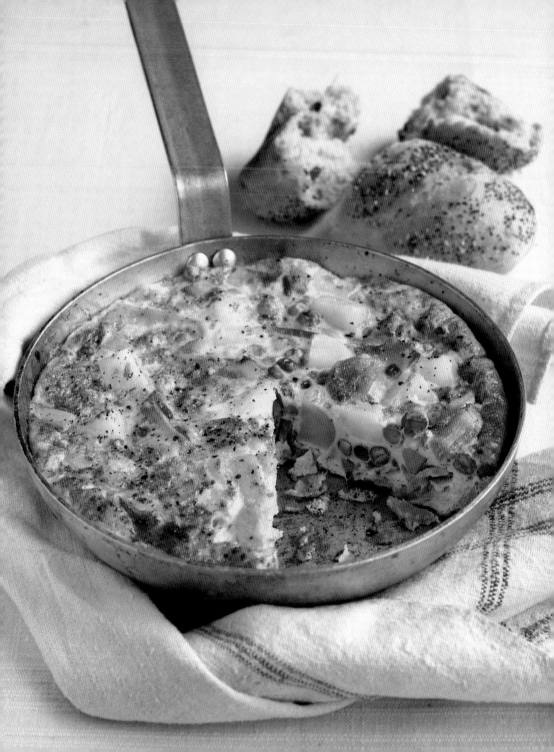

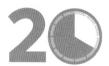

Veggie Noodles with Hoi Sin

Serves 4

175 g (6 oz) egg noodles

4 tablespoons sesame oil

200 g (7 oz) baby corn, roughly chopped

1 large red pepper, cut into strips

bunch of spring onions, roughly chopped

200 g (7 oz) green beans, roughly chopped

2.5 cm (1 inch) piece of fresh root ginger, peeled and grated

1 garlic clove, crushed

4 tablespoons clear honey

1 tablespoon dark soy sauce

4 tablespoons sweet chilli sauce

4 tablespoons toasted sesame seeds

- Cook the noodles in a large saucepan of lightly salted boiling water for 8–10 minutes or according to the packet instructions.

- Meanwhile, heat the oil in a large heavy-based frying pan. Add the baby corn and red pepper over a high heat for 3 minutes, stirring occasionally. Add the spring onions, sugarsnap peas, ginger and garlic and stir-fry for 4 minutes until softened, but not too golden – reduce the heat if they start to brown.

- Drain the noodles, add to the frying pan and toss. Mix together the honey, soy sauce, sweet chilli and sesame seeds, pour over the noodles and toss again for 1 minute until hot. Serve in warmed serving bowls.

Cheat's Veggie Noodles

Heat 2 tablespoons sesame oil in a large wok or frying pan and stir-fry 400 g (13 oz) ready-prepared 'family stir-fry' veg for 3–4 minutes until tender but retaining their shape. In a separate pan, heat 2 tablespoons sesame oil and stir-fry 250 g (8 oz) straight-to-wok egg noodles for 2–3 minutes until separated and hot. Toss into the veg, add 1 tablespoon dark soy sauce and 2 tablespoons sweet chilli sauce and toss. Scatter with 2 tablespoons toasted sesame seeds, toss again and serve.

Vegetable and Egg Noodles

Cook 250 g (8 oz) soba noodles in a saucepan of lightly salted boiling water for 10 minutes until tender, then drain. Meanwhile, heat 2 tablespoons sesame oil in a large wok or frying pan. Break in 2 beaten eggs, cook over a medium heat for 2 minutes until golden and set, then flip over and cook for a further 30 seconds until golden. Remove from the pan and roughly chop, then set aside. Heat a further 2 tablespoons sesame oil in the wok or frying pan and cook 200 g (7 oz) baby corn, cut in half lengthways, and 1 large red pepper, cut into strips, for 5 minutes. Add a bunch of roughly chopped spring onions, 200 g (7 oz) roughly chopped sugarsnap peas, a 2.5 cm (1 inch) piece of fresh root ginger, peeled and grated, and 1 garlic clove, crushed, and stir-fry for a further 3–4 minutes. Add the drained noodles and stir-fry for 2 minutes, add the egg and toss. Serve hot in warmed serving bowls scattered with 2 tablespoons toasted sesame seeds, with soy sauce or chilli sauce drizzled over, if liked.

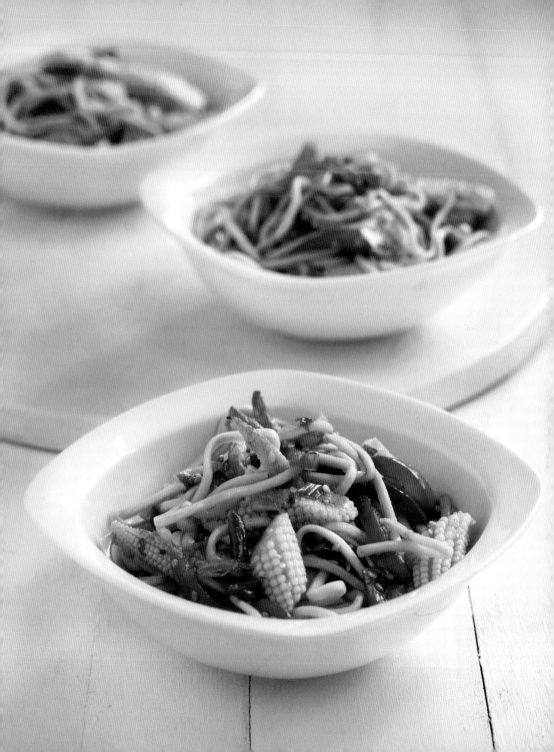

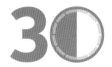

30 Potato Skins with Homemade Guacamole

Serves 4

6 baking potatoes, washed
4 tablespoons olive oil
1 teaspoon Cajun spice
1 avocado, halved, peeled and
   stoned
finely grated rind and juice of
   ½ lemon
1 tablespoon sweet chilli sauce
2 tablespoons finely chopped
   coriander
pepper

- Prick the potatoes all over and cook for 10 minutes in a microwave on full power. Remove from the microwave, cut each in half and scoop out most of the potato, leaving a 1 cm (½ inch) border of potato next to the skin. Discard the potato (or keep for mashed potato for another recipe).

- Cut each half into 2 wedges and place on a baking sheet. Mix the oil with the Cajun spice and brush over the potato skins on both sides. Place on a baking sheet and cook under a preheated grill for 5–7 minutes, then turn the skins over and cook for a further 5–7 minutes until crisp and golden.

- Meanwhile, mash the avocado with the lemon rind and juice, season with pepper and mix in the chilli sauce and coriander. Transfer to a small serving bowl and put it on a serving platter. Place the hot potato skins on the platter and use them to dip into the guacamole.

---

10 Pan-Fried Potato Cakes with Guacamole Divide 300 g (10 oz) chilled ready-made mashed potato into 4. Shape each piece of mash into 4 patty shapes and toss in seasoned flour. Heat 4 tablespoons vegetable oil in a large heavy-based frying pan and cook the potato cakes over a high heat for 4 minutes on each side until golden. Serve hot with spoonfuls of chilled ready-made guacamole and scatter with 2 finely chopped spring onions to serve.

20 Potato Wedges with Guacamole Place 450 g (14½ oz) ready-prepared herby potato wedges in a roasting tin. Cook under a preheated grill for 8–10 minutes until golden, then turn them over using a fish slice and cook for a further 6–8 minutes until golden and crisp. Meanwhile, make the guacamole. Mash 1 peeled, stoned ripe avocado with the finely grated rind and juice of 1 lemon, then stir in 1 tablespoon sweet chilli sauce and 2 tablespoons chopped coriander.

Serve the hot wedges scattered with 2 finely chopped spring onions ready to dip in the guacamole.

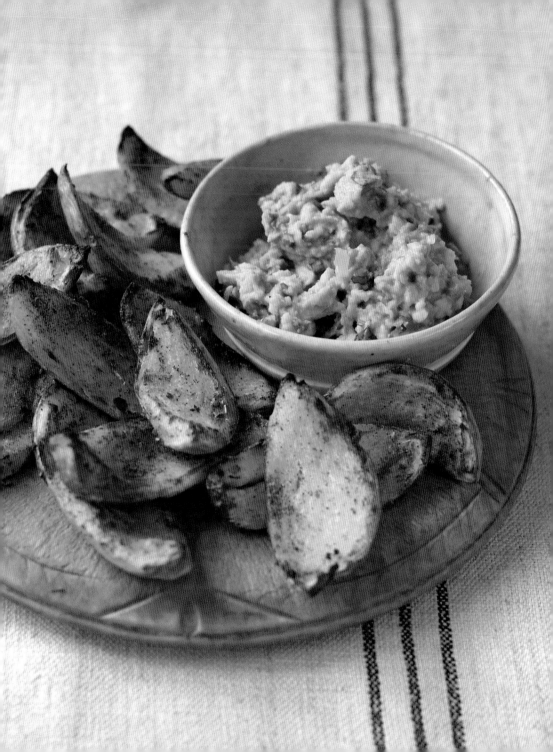

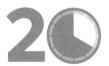 # Tomato and Spinach Ravioli Gratin

Serves 4

300 g (10 oz) spinach and ricotta
  ravioli
3 tablespoons olive oil
250 g (8 oz) cherry plum
  tomatoes
2 x 400 g (13 oz) cans chopped
  tomatoes
3 tablespoons sun-dried tomato
  paste
175 g (6 oz) baby spinach leaves
150 g (5 oz) mozzarella cheese,
  drained and thinly sliced
4 tablespoons grated Parmesan
  cheese
pepper

To serve
garlic bread
salad

- Cook the ravioli in a large saucepan of lightly salted boiling water for 3 minutes or according to the packet instructions, then drain.

- Meanwhile, heat the oil in a large heavy-based frying pan, add the cherry plum tomatoes to the pan and cook for 3–4 minutes until beginning to soften and 'pop'. Add the chopped tomatoes and sun-dried tomato paste and bring to the boil, then add the baby spinach leaves and cook and stir for 3–4 minutes until all the ingredients are piping hot and the spinach has wilted. Season generously with pepper.

- Add the drained pasta to the pan and toss well, then transfer to a shallow gratin dish. Arrange the mozzarella slices over the pasta, then scatter over the Parmesan.

- Cook under a preheated grill for 3–4 minutes until golden and bubbling. Serve with garlic bread and salad.

 Spinach Ravioli with Tomato Sauce

Cook 300 g (10 oz) spinach and ricotta ravioli in lightly salted boiling water for 3 minutes, then drain. Meanwhile, heat 1 tablespoon olive oil in a frying pan and cook 175 g (6 oz) cherry tomatoes over a high heat for 2 minutes. Add 400 ml (14 fl oz) passata and 2 tablespoons sun-dried tomato paste, bring to the boil and cook for 2 minutes. Add the ravioli and toss well. Serve scattered with grated Parmesan cheese.

Spinach and Ricotta Cannelloni with Tomato Sauce Place 300 g (10 oz) washed spinach leaves in a saucepan with 1 tablespoon cold water and cook over a medium heat, stirring occasionally, until wilted. Remove from the heat, transfer to a colander and squeeze out as much water as possible, then place in a mixing bowl with 250 g (8 oz) ricotta cheese and 1 teaspoon ground nutmeg. Mix well and season with pepper. Take 4 large lasagne sheets and divide the ricotta and spinach mixture between them down the centre lengthways. Roll up the lasagne sheets to enclose the filling and place the 'tubes' in a rectangular shallow gratin dish. Pour over 300 ml (½ pint) ready-made tomato pasta sauce and scatter with 2 tablespoons grated Parmesan cheese. Bake in a preheated oven, 220°C (425°F), Gas Mark 7, for 15 minutes until piping hot. Serve with garlic bread and salad.

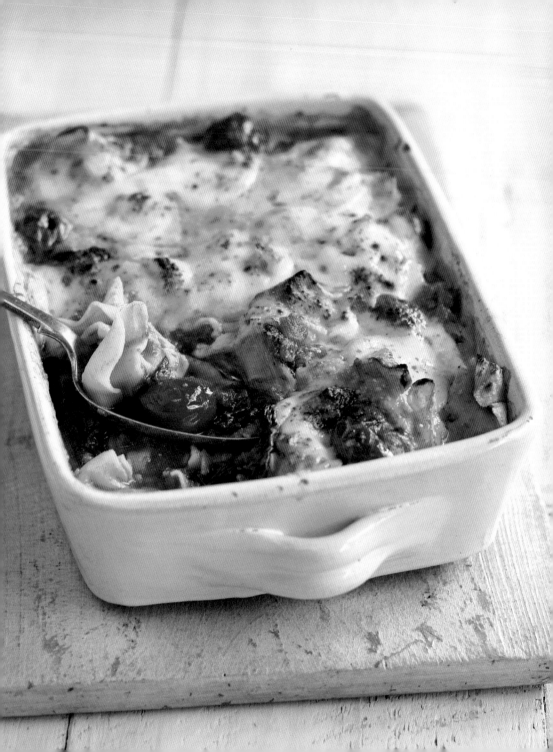

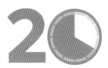

Chicken, Pesto and Bacon Pan-Fry

Serves 4

4 small chicken breasts, about
150 g (5 oz) each
4 tablespoons pesto
4 good-quality back bacon
rashers
2 tablespoons olive oil

To serve

seasonal vegetables
new potatoes (optional)

- Make a slit in each chicken breast along its length. Open and fill with the pesto. Stretch each bacon rasher with the back of a sharp knife to lengthen, then wrap tightly around the chicken breast to enclose the pesto filling.

- Heat the oil in a large heavy-based frying pan and cook the chicken breasts over a medium-high heat for 10–12 minutes until golden and cooked through.

- Serve the chicken with seasonal vegetables and new potatoes, if liked.

Chicken, Bacon and Pesto Stir-Fry

Heat 2 tablespoons olive oil in a wok or large heavy-based frying pan and stir-fry 375 g (12 oz) chicken mini-fillets over a high heat for 3–4 minutes. Add 6 roughly chopped bacon rashers and cook for a further 3 minutes until golden. Add 175 g (6 oz) halved cherry tomatoes and stir-fry for a further 2 minutes, then add 2 tablespoons pesto and heat for 1 minute until piping hot. Serve with warm crusty bread.

Chicken and Pesto Burgers With

Bacon Put 500 g (1 lb) minced chicken in a food processor with 2 tablespoons pesto, season with pepper and whizz briefly to blend together. Shape the mixture, using hands lightly coated with flour (or cornmeal), into 4 patties and set aside. Heat 3 tablespoons olive oil in a large heavy-based frying pan and cook the burgers over a high heat for 7–8 minutes on each side until golden and cooked through. Meanwhile, cook 4 back bacon rashers under a preheated grill for 4–5 minutes until golden and cooked. Serve the burgers in wholemeal buns with a spoonful of ready-made béarnaise sauce on each and topped with a bacon rasher. Top with rocket or the children's favourite salad leaves and serve.

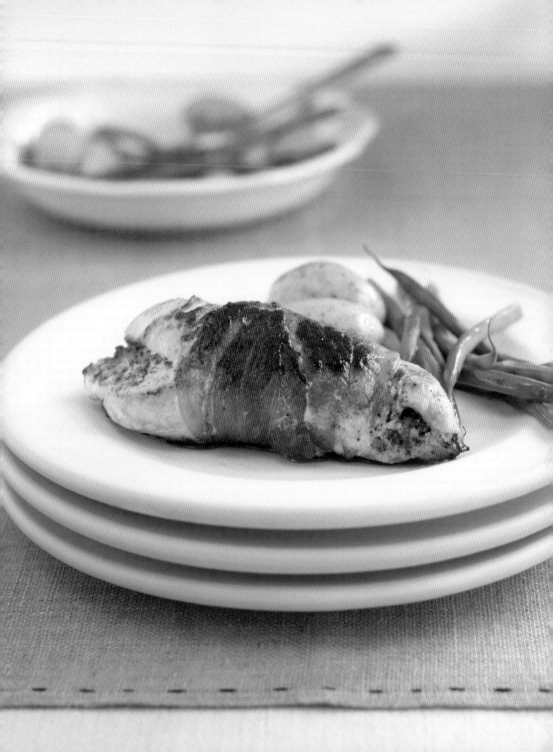

30 Spaghetti Bolognese

Serves 4

250 g (8 oz) spaghetti
2 tablespoons olive oil
1 onion, finely chopped
2 garlic cloves, crushed
1 large carrot, peeled and finely chopped
75 g (3 oz) mushrooms, roughly chopped
1 teaspoon dried oregano
½ teaspoon dried thyme
375 g (12 oz) good-quality minced beef
300 ml (½ pint) beef stock
300 ml (½ pint) passata
grated Parmesan cheese, to serve

- Bring a large pan of lightly salted water to the boil, cook the spaghetti for 15–20 minutes until tender, then drain and keep warm.

- Meanwhile, heat the oil in a large heavy-based saucepan. Add the onion and cook over a high heat for 2–3 minutes, then add the garlic, carrot and mushrooms and cook for 5 minutes. Add the herbs and mince and cook for 10 minutes until the meat is golden. Add the stock and passata and continue to cook for a further 10 minutes, stirring occasionally, until the sauce has thickened and the meat and vegetables are tender and cooked through.

- Add the spaghetti to the pan, mix with the meat and vegetables and serve piled into warm serving bowls with the grated Parmesan on top.

 Bolognese Ravioli with Tomato Sauce

Cook 350 g (11½ oz) bolognese ravioli in lightly salted boiling water for 3 minutes. Meanwhile, heat 2 tablespoons olive oil in a pan and cook 8 roughly chopped tomatoes and 1 crushed clove garlic for 3 minutes, stirring continuously. Add 2 tablespoons tomato purée and 150 ml (¼ pint) vegetable stock and bring to the boil. Transfer to a food processor and whizz until smooth. Toss into the drained pasta in a pan and stir. Serve in warmed bowls scattered with grated Parmesan cheese.

 Fusilli Bolognese Gratin

Cook 500 g (1 lb) fusilli pasta in a large pan of lightly salted boiling water, for 3 minutes, then drain and set aside. Meanwhile, heat a large frying pan and cook 375 g (12 oz) good-quality minced beef for 10 minutes, stirring occasionally, until well browned. Add 400 ml (14 fl oz) ready-made bolognese tomato sauce and 6 tablespoons chopped basil. Cover and simmer for 5 minutes. Add the drained pasta, transfer to a shallow gratin dish and scatter with 6 tablespoons grated Parmesan cheese.

Cook under a preheated grill for 2–3 minutes until golden and bubbling, then serve with salad and garlic bread.

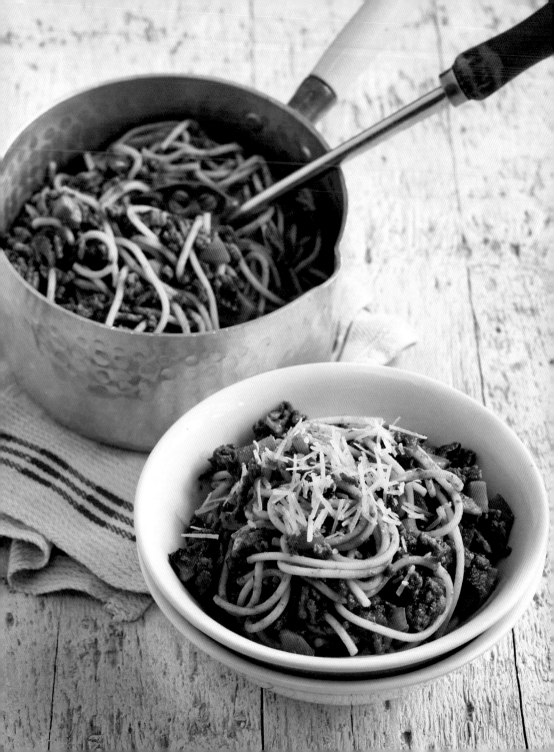

1 0 Frankfurter and Courgette Frittata

Serves 4

2 tablespoons olive oil

1 large courgette, cut into small chunks

6 frankfurters, chopped

6 eggs, beaten

100 g (3½ oz) feta cheese, crumbled

pepper

salad, to serve

- Heat the oil in a medium nonstick frying pan. Add the courgette and frankfurters and fry, stirring, for 3 minutes until the courgette has softened.

- Season the eggs with pepper (there is no need to add salt as the feta is quite salty). Pour into the pan and cook, stirring gently, until the mixture starts to set. Scatter over the feta cheese.

- Place the pan under a preheated hot grill keeping the handle away from the heat, and cook for 1 minute until the top is set. Cut into wedges and serve with salad.

2 0 Frankfurter and Courgette Omelette

Heat 2 tablespoons olive oil in a nonstick frying pan, add 1 chopped onion and 1 chopped courgette and fry, stirring occasionally, for 5 minutes until the onion has softened and is starting to brown. Add 4 chopped frankfurters and fry for 2 minutes. Lightly beat 6 eggs and season with pepper. Pour into the pan and scatter over 4 halved cherry tomatoes and 200 g (7 oz) crumbled feta cheese. Cook the omelette, stirring lightly, until most of the egg has set. Carefully turn the omelette out of the pan, then slide it back in to cook the other side. Serve cut into wedges with peas.

3 0 Simple Frankfurter and Courgette Quiche

Fry 1 chopped courgette in 2 tablespoons olive oil for 3 minutes until softened and just starting to brown. Scatter over the base of a ready-made savoury pastry case with 4 chopped frankfurters and 200 g (7 oz) crumbled feta cheese. Mix together 4 beaten eggs and 150 ml (¼ pint) single cream. Season lightly with pepper and pour over the filling in the pastry case. Bake in a preheated oven, 200°C (400°F), Gas Mark 6, for 20 minutes until the filling has just set.

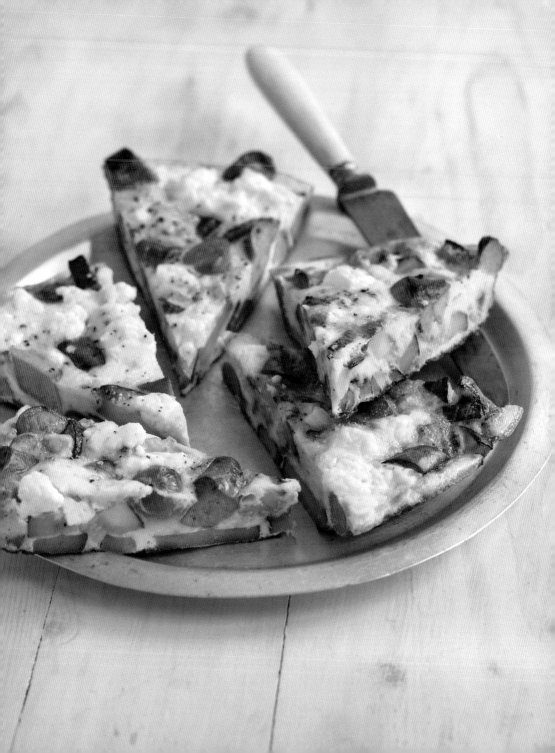

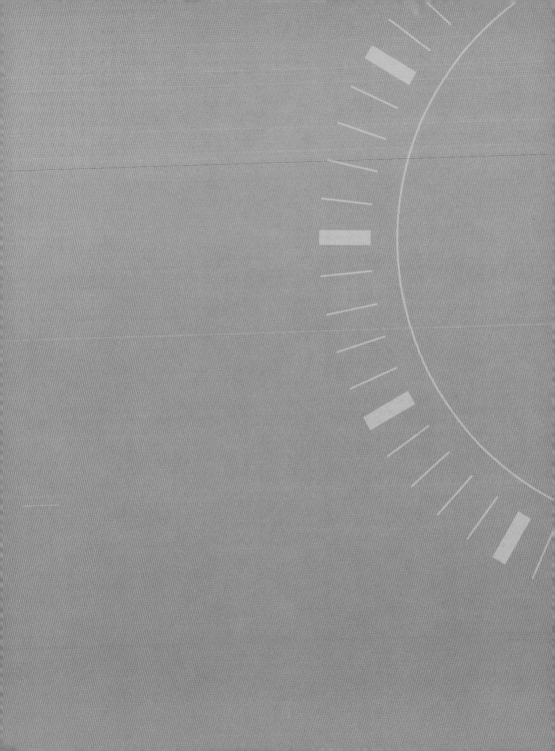

QuickCook
For All The Family

Recipes listed by cooking time

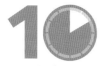

Curried Chicken, Mango and Coconut Stir-Fry

Serves 4

1 tablespoon oil
350 g (11½ oz) chicken mini-
   fillets, roughly chopped
250 g (8 oz) ready-prepared
   freshly mango pieces
2 teaspoons curry powder
400 g (13 oz) ready-prepared
   mixed stir-fry vegetables
200 ml (7 fl oz) coconut milk

To serve

mango chutney (optional)
wholemeal chapattis (optional)

- Heat the oil in a large heavy-based frying pan and fry the chicken over a high heat for 4–5 minutes until golden and cooked through. Add the mango and curry powder and stir-fry for a further minute.

- Add the stir-fry vegetables and cook over a high heat for 3 minutes until the vegetables are just tender, but still retaining their shape. Add the coconut milk and heat for 1 minute until piping hot.

- Serve with mango chutney and wholemeal chapattis, if liked.

 Coconuty Chicken and Mango Korma

Heat 1 tablespoon oil in a heavy-based frying pan and cook 375 g (12 oz) chicken breast pieces and 1 small finely chopped onion for 7–8 minutes until golden. Add 2 tablespoons korma curry paste and cook for 1 minute. Add 1 mango, cut into chunks, and cook for 1 minute, stirring. Add a 400 ml (14 fl oz) can coconut milk and 150 ml (¼ pint) chicken stock and bring to the boil. Reduce the heat and simmer for 5 minutes. Meanwhile, blend 2 teaspoons cornflour with 2 tablespoons water. Add to the curry and stir until thick. Add 4 tablespoons chopped coriander and serve with warm naan, rice or chapatti.

 Chicken, Mango and Coconut Biryani Cook 200 g (7 oz) wholemeal rice in a large saucepan of lightly salted boiling water for 20–25 minutes until tender, adding 125 g (4 oz) frozen peas for the final 5 minutes of cooking. Heat 2 tablespoons oil in a large heavy-based frying pan and cook 250 g (8 oz) roughly chopped chicken mini-fillets and 1 sliced onion for 7–8 minutes until golden and cooked through. Add 2 tablespoons korma curry paste and stir, then add a 400 ml (14 fl oz) can coconut milk and bring to the boil. Reduce the heat, cover and simmer for 10 minutes, stirring occasionally, until the coconut milk has

reduced by half. For the final 2 minutes, add 250 g (8 oz) ready-prepared fresh mango pieces. Drain the rice and peas, add to the pan with 6 tablespoons chopped coriander and toss well. Serve in warmed serving bowls.

KID-FORA-QOU

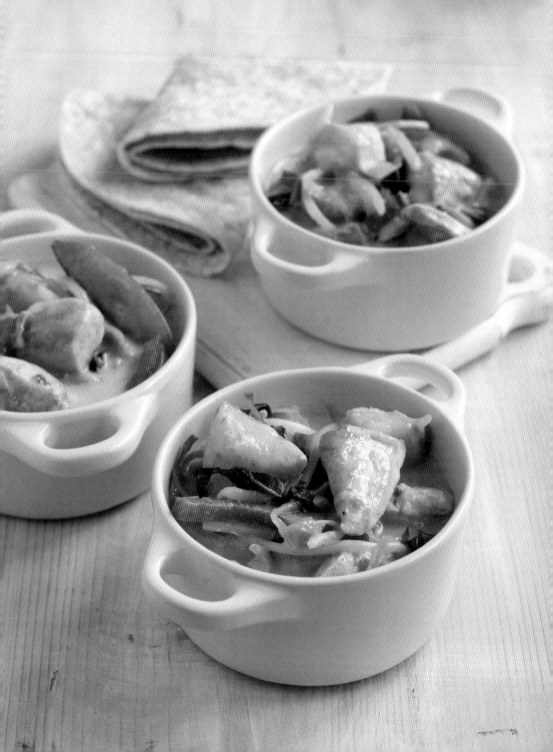

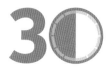 # Cheesy Pesto Baked Potatoes

Serves 4

4 small/medium baking potatoes
125 g (4 oz) spinach leaves
1 tablespoon water
2 tablespoons pesto
4 tablespoons grated Parmesan
   cheese
pepper
baked beans, to serve

- Place the potatoes on a microwave-proof plate and pierce several times with a sharp knife, then cook for 5 minutes in a microwave. Turn and cook again for a further 3 minutes, then transfer to the top of a preheated oven, 220°C (425°F), Gas Mark 7, for 5 minutes to golden a little.

- Meanwhile, place the spinach in a saucepan with the measurement water and heat over a medium heat for 5 minutes until wilted.

- Remove the potatoes from the oven, cut in half lengthways and scoop out most of the flesh, reserving the skins. Put the potato into a bowl and season with pepper. Mash and stir with the pesto, then fold in the spinach leaves.

- Place the potato halves on a baking sheet, pile the pesto potato back into the skins and scatter with the Parmesan. Cook under a preheated grill for 5 minutes until golden and bubbling. Serve with baked beans.

 Cheesy Pesto Mash Mix 500 g (1 lb) chilled ready-made mashed potato with 2 tablespoons pesto, 3 tablespoons grated Parmesan cheese and 1 egg. Heat 15 g (½ oz) butter in a nonstick frying pan, press the potato mixture into the base and cook over a medium heat for 4 minutes. Scatter over 2 tablespoons grated Parmesan and place the pan under a preheated grill (keeping the handle away from the heat) and cook for 2 minutes until golden. Serve in wedges.

Cheesy Potato and Pesto Hash Pierce the top of a 400 g (13 oz) pack of potato wedges with herbs and pierce the top a few times, then microwave for 8–10 minutes until tender. Heat 3 tablespoons vegetable oil in a nonstick frying pan and cook 1 chopped onion for 2 minutes. Roughly chop the cooked potatoes, add to the onion and cook for 5 minutes, stirring occasionally, until golden and crisp in places. Add 2 tablespoons pesto, stir and cook for a further 2–3 minutes. Remove from the heat and scatter with 4 tablespoons grated Parmesan cheese. Place the pan under a preheated grill (keeping the handle away from the heat) and cook for 2–3 minutes until golden and bubbling. Serve hot.

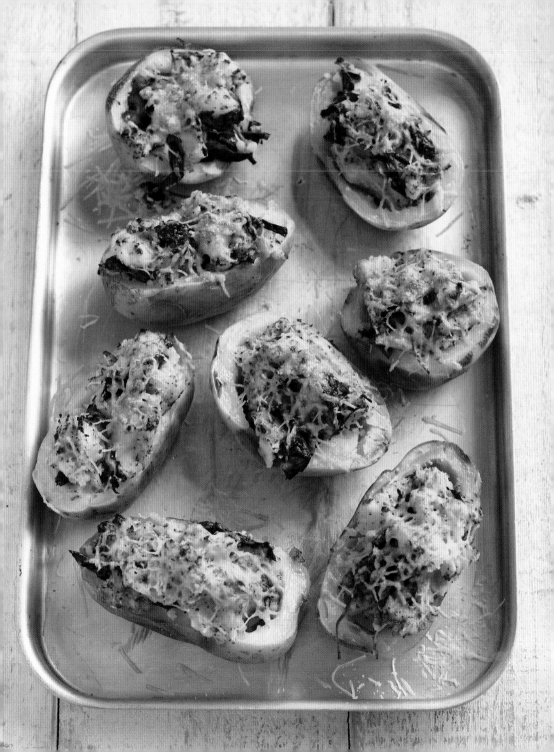

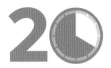

Rosti with Bacon and Mushrooms

Serves 4

500 g (1 lb) potatoes, peeled and
coarsely grated

1 parsnip, peeled and coarsely
grated

25 g (1 oz) butter

2 tablespoons sunflower oil

8 bacon rashers

150 g (5 oz) chestnut
mushrooms, halved, if large

salt and pepper

To serve

baked beans

tomato ketchup

- Squeeze out any moisture from the grated potatoes and parsnips. Mix together in a bowl and season with salt and pepper. Heat the butter and 1 tablespoon of the oil in a large nonstick frying pan. When the butter is melted and foaming, add the potato mixture and spread out evenly. Cook over a medium heat for about 5 minutes until the base is golden and crisp.

- Place a large plate or baking sheet over the pan and turn the rosti out. Slide it back into the pan and cook for about 10 minutes until the potato and parsnip are tender and golden.

- Meanwhile, heat the remaining oil in a separate frying pan. Add the bacon and mushrooms and fry for 5 minutes until the bacon is crisp and the mushrooms are tender.

- Cut the rosti cake into wedges and serve with the bacon, mushrooms, baked beans and ketchup.

Bacon and Mushroom Hash

Drain 575 g (1¼ lb) canned new potatoes and cut into quarters. Cook in a large frying pan with 2 tablespoons sunflower oil, 4 chopped bacon rashers and 150 g (5 oz) halved mushrooms for 5 minutes until golden. Add a sprinkle of Cajun seasoning and a handful of frozen peas. Cook, stirring, for a few minutes until the peas are hot. Serve with crème fraîche and crusty bread.

Bacon Bubble and Squeak

Cook 500 g (1 lb) peeled and chopped potatoes in lightly salted boiling water for 10 minutes until tender. Drain and mash with 25 g (1 oz) butter, a dash of milk and salt and pepper. Cook 375 g (12 oz) mixed frozen vegetables, drain and roughly mash. (Alternatively, use any leftover mash and vegetables you may have.) Stir the vegetables into the mash.

Cook 4 chopped bacon rashers in a large nonstick frying pan for 3 minutes until crisp. Remove the bacon from the pan and stir into the potato mixture. Add 2 tablespoons sunflower oil to the bacon fat in the pan and heat. Spoon in the potato mixture and spread evenly. Cook for 5 minutes until golden and crisp underneath, then turn over and cook for a further 5–10 minutes. Serve in wedges topped with fried eggs.

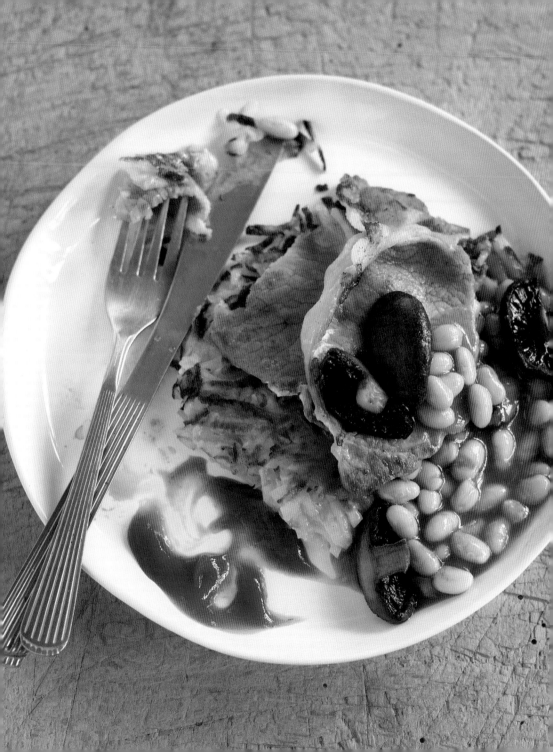

Hearty Bean, Bacon and Pasta Soup

Serves 4

2 tablespoons olive oil

125 g (4 oz) bacon, roughly snipped

1 small onion, roughly chopped

1 celery stick

1 carrot, peeled and roughly chopped

2 x 400 g (13 oz) cans mixed beans, rinsed and drained

2 tablespoons tomato purée

600 ml (1 pint) chicken stock

125 g (4 oz) pasta shapes

To serve

grated Parmesan cheese

chopped parsley, (optional)

warm crusty bread

- Heat the oil in a large heavy-based saucepan and cook the bacon, onion, celery and carrot for 5 minutes. Add the beans, tomato purée and stock and bring to the boil. Reduce the heat and simmer for 10 minutes.

- Cook the pasta shapes in a small saucepan of lightly salted boiling water for 8–10 minutes until tender. Drain and set aside.

- Place the bean and stock mixture in a food processor and whizz until smooth. Return to the pan, add the pasta and heat for 1 minute. Ladle into serving bowls and sprinkle with Parmesan and parsley, if liked. Serve with warm crusty bread.

 Quick Bean Soup with Crispy Bacon

Place a 400 g (13 oz) can mixed beans, rinsed and drained, into a food processor with a 400 g (13 oz) can chopped tomatoes and whizz until smooth. Transfer to a large heavy-based saucepan with 2 tablespoons tomato purée and 300 ml (½ pint) chicken stock and bring to the boil. Season well and ladle into soup bowls. Serve scattered with 1 tablespoon ready-made croutons and some crispy bacon bits.

 Bean and Bacon Pasta Gratin

Heat 2 tablespoons olive oil in a large frying pan and cook 125 g (4 oz) roughly chopped bacon, 1 small roughly chopped onion, 1 celery stick and 1 peeled and roughly chopped carrot over a medium heat for 5 minutes until softened. Add a 400 g (13 oz) can mixed beans, rinsed and drained, a 400 g (13 oz) can chopped tomatoes and 1 tablespoon tomato purée. Bring to the boil, stirring, then remove from the heat. Meanwhile, cook 250 g (8 oz) pasta shells in a large saucepan of lightly salted boiling water for 8–10 minutes until tender. Drain, add to the bacon and beans and stir and toss well. Transfer to a large gratin dish, sprinkle with 125 g (4 oz) grated Cheddar cheese and cook under a preheated hot grill for 5 minutes until golden and bubbling. Serve hot with crusty bread and salad.

KID-FORA-PIQ

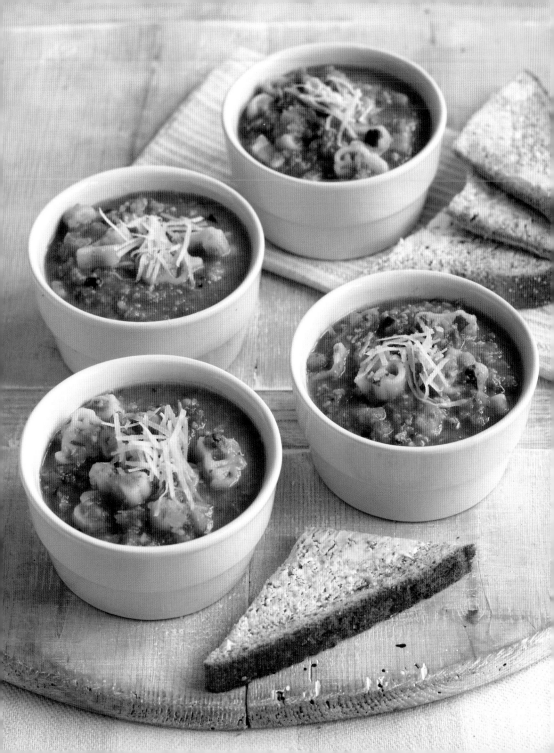

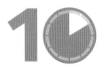

Kedgeree-Style Rice with Spinach

Serves 4

250 g (8 oz) smoked haddock fillets

125 g (4 oz) frozen peas

150 ml (¼ pint) boiling water

250 g (8 oz) spinach leaves

500 g (1 lb) express rice

25 g (1 oz) butter

½ teaspoon garam masala

pepper

3 tablespoons chopped parsley, to garnish (optional)

- Place the haddock and peas in a frying pan, cover with the measurement water and bring to the boil. Reduce the heat, cover and simmer for 3–4 minutes, adding the spinach for the final minute of cooking.

- Meanwhile, microwave the express rice for 5 minutes or according to the packet instructions. Drain the fish, spinach and peas and flake the fish. Return to the pan and add the butter, garam masala and rice, season with pepper and toss well.

- Serve sprinkled with parsley, if liked.

 Classic Kedgeree with Spinach

Cook 250 g (8 oz) easy-cook basmati rice and 4 eggs in a saucepan of lightly salted boiling water for 15 minutes until the rice is tender, adding the peas for the final 5 minutes. Meanwhile, place 250 g (8 oz) smoked haddock or cod fillets in a frying pan, pour over about 150 ml (¼ pint) water, cover with a tight-fitting lid and bring to the boil. Cook for 5 minutes until the fish is opaque and cooked through. Meanwhile, heat 2 tablespoons oil in a large heavy-based frying pan and cook 1 chopped onion over a medium heat for 3–4 minutes. Add 2 tablespoons garam masala and cook for 1 minute, stirring, then add 200 g (7 oz) spinach leaves, toss and cook for 2–3 minutes until the spinach has wilted. Drain the rice, removing the eggs. Add the rice and peas to the onion mixture and toss over the heat. Drain and flake the fish, add to the rice and toss well. Shell the eggs and roughly chop, then add to the rice and toss again. Serve on warmed serving plates.

 Creamy Haddock and Spinach

Risotto Heat 2 tablespoons olive oil in a pan and cook 1 chopped onion for 3–4 minutes, then add 250 g (8 oz) Arborio rice and 1 teaspoon garam masala and stir to coat in oil. Pour in 600 ml (1 pint) fish stock, bring to the boil, reduce the heat and simmer for 10 minutes until the stock is absorbed. Add 450 ml (¾ pint) fish stock, cover and simmer for 2 minutes. Stir in 250 g (8 oz) roughly chopped smoked haddock fillets, 125 g (4 oz) frozen peas and 200 g (7 oz) spinach. Increase the heat and cook for 5 minutes until the fish is opaque and cooked. Season with pepper, stir in 200 ml (7 fl oz) crème fraîche and heat for 2–3 minutes, stirring until hot. Serve with crusty bread.

KID-FORA-SYC

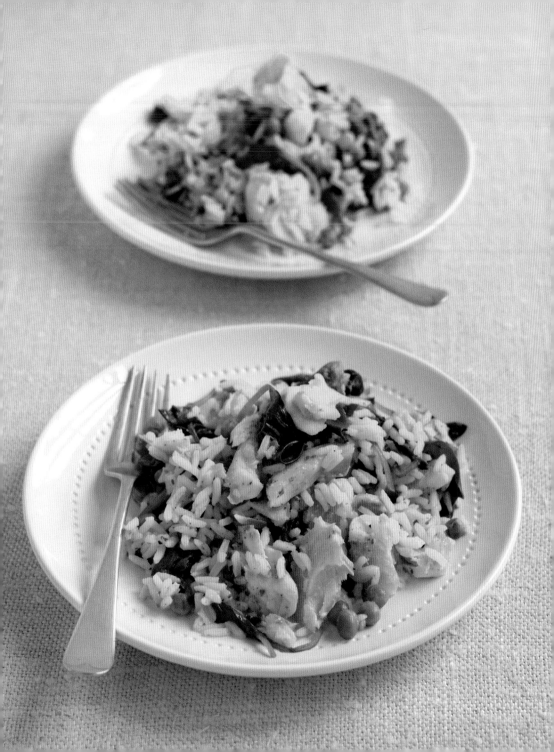

30 Warm Mozzarella, Chicken, Tomato and Basil Pasta

Serves 4

250 g (8 oz) penne

4 tablespoons olive oil

250 g (8 oz) chicken breast, cut into strips

4 tablespoons pine nuts

150 g (5 oz) cherry tomatoes, halved

6 tablespoons chopped basil leaves

125 g (4 oz) baby mozzarella balls, drained

pepper

- Cook the penne in a large saucepan of lightly salted boiling water for 10–12 minutes until tender. Drain and keep warm.

- Meanwhile, heat the oil in a large heavy-based frying pan and cook the chicken over a high heat for 8–10 minutes until golden and cooked through. Add the pine nuts and cook for a further 2 minutes until golden. Add the cherry tomato halves and toss and cook for a further 2 minutes.

- Add the drained pasta to the pan and toss well, then stir in the chopped basil and season well with pepper.

- Turn into a serving bowl and stir in the mozzarella balls.

 Cheese-Filled Pasta with Tomatoes and Basil Cook 300 g (10 oz) 3-cheese-filled pasta in a saucepan of lightly salted boiling water for 3–4 minutes. Meanwhile, heat 3 tablespoons olive oil in a frying pan and cook 4 tablespoons pine nuts for 1 minute, then add 175 g (6 oz) halved cherry tomatoes and cook for 2–3 minutes until softened but retaining their shape. Drain the pasta, toss into the pan with the tomatoes and pine nuts and stir well. Transfer to warmed serving bowls and scatter with basil leaves.

 Cheesy Tomato and Basil Pasta Melt Cook 250 g (8 oz) pasta shapes in a large pan of lightly salted boiling water for 10 minutes until tender. Drain and keep warm. Heat 1 tablespoon olive oil in a large frying pan and cook 4 tablespoons pine nuts for 1 minute, then add 375 g (12 oz) whole cherry tomatoes over a high heat for 2–3 minutes until the tomatoes have softened. Add the drained pasta to the pan and toss well, then add 8 tablespoons chopped basil leaves and season well with pepper. Arrange in a medium gratin dish, then top with 300 g (10 oz) sliced mozzarella cheese. Cook under a preheated medium grill for 3–4 minutes until golden and bubbling.

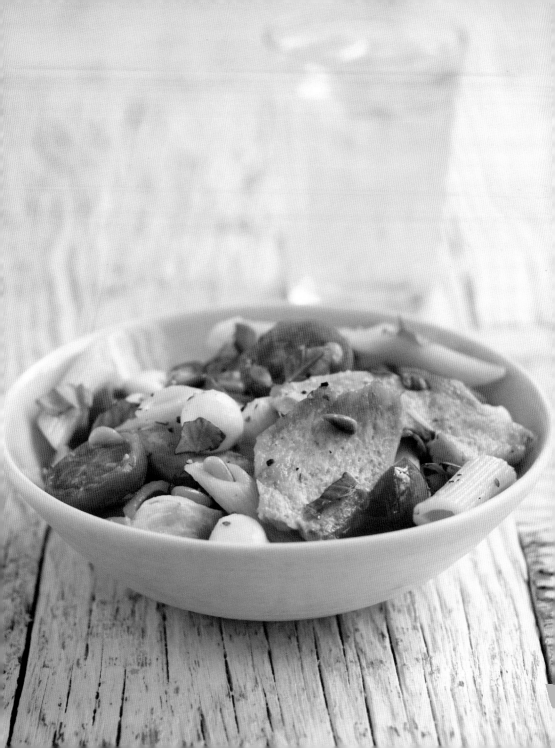

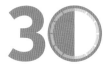

30 Creamy Mushroom Pork and Apple Pies

Serves 4

1 kg (2 lb) potatoes, peeled and chopped
1 tablespoon sunflower oil
1 onion, chopped
450 g (14½ oz) pork steaks, cut into bite-sized pieces
1 dessert apple, peeled, cored and chopped
150 g (5 oz) sliced mushrooms
200 ml (7 fl oz) crème fraîche
100 ml (3½ fl oz) chicken stock
1 teaspoon Dijon mustard
25 g (1 oz) butter
4 tablespoons milk
50 g (2 oz) Cheddar cheese, grated
salt and pepper
peas, to serve
cherry tomatoes, basil leaves and chives, to garnish

- Cook the potatoes in a large saucepan of lightly salted boiling water for 10–15 minutes until tender.

- Meanwhile, heat the oil in a frying pan. Add the onion and pork and fry over a high heat for 5 minutes, stirring occasionally. Add the apple and mushrooms and cook for a further 2 minutes. Stir in the crème fraîche, stock and mustard and season with salt and pepper. Simmer for 5 minutes.

- When the potatoes are cooked, drain and mash with the butter and milk and season with salt and pepper. Spoon the pork mixture into individual flameproof dishes and spoon the mash over the top. Make ridges in the mash with the back of a fork and sprinkle the cheese over the top. Cook under a preheated medium grill until the cheese melts.

- Garnish the pies with animal faces using cherry tomatoes for noses, peas for eyes, basil leaves for ears and chives for whiskers. Serve with peas.

 Creamy Mushroom Pork and Apple

Cook a garlic baguette in a preheated oven, 220°C (450°F), Gas Mark 7, for 10 minutes. Meanwhile, fry 4 thin pork steaks, about 125 g (4 oz) each, for 3 minutes, turning once. Add 1 sliced apple, cook for 1 minute, then stir in 350 g (11½ oz) ready-made mushroom pasta sauce. Bring to the boil and simmer for 5 minutes. Serve with the garlic bread.

 Curried Pork and Apple Filo Pies

Cut 400 g (13 oz) pork steaks into small chunks and fry in 1 tablespoon sunflower oil for 5 minutes until browned and just cooked. Stir in 2 tablespoons korma curry paste, fry for 1 minute, then add a 400 ml (14 oz) can coconut milk. Bring to the boil, reduce the heat and simmer for 5 minutes. Stir in 1 chopped dessert apple, 50 g (2 oz) sultanas and 2 tablespoons chopped coriander. Brush 4 sheets of filo pastry with 50 g (2 oz) melted butter and ruffle to make 4 scrunched rounds to fit the tops of 4 individual pie dishes. Spoon the curry into dishes. Place the filo on top, sprinkle with sesame seeds and bake in a preheated oven, 220°C (450°F), Gas Mark 7, for 10 minutes until the pastry is golden. Serve with green beans.

KID-FORA-WYA

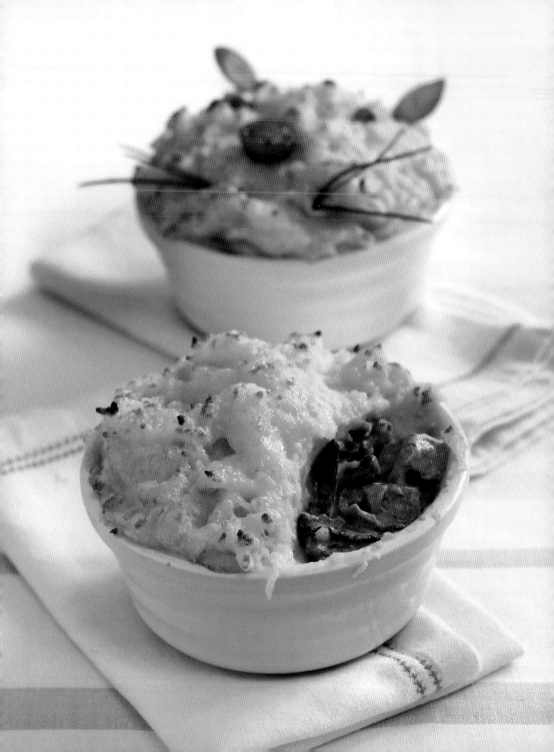

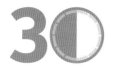

Spiced Rice and Chickpea Balls with Sweet Chilli Sauce

Serves 4

75 g (3 oz) Arborio risotto rice
300 ml (½ pint) vegetable stock
1 teaspoon minced garlic
1 teaspoon ground cumin
1 teaspoon ground coriander
½ teaspoon paprika
¼ teaspoon turmeric
3 tablespoons chopped coriander
400 g (13 oz) can chickpeas, rinsed and drained
1 egg yolk
125 g (4 oz) cornmeal or polenta
5 tablespoons sesame seeds
4 tablespoons vegetable oil
pepper
sweet chilli sauce, to serve

- Place the rice in a small saucepan with the stock and bring to the boil. Reduce the heat, cover and simmer for 15 minutes until the rice is tender and sticky. Stir in the garlic, spices and chopped coriander.

- Meanwhile, put the chickpeas in a food processor and whizz until almost smooth, but still retaining some texture. Add the cooked sticky rice to the bowl with the egg yolk and whizz together, then season with pepper.

- Mix together the cornmeal or polenta and sesame seeds in a bowl. Form the chickpea mixture into walnut-sized balls and coat in the cornmeal mixture. Heat the oil in a large heavy-based frying pan and cook over a high heat for 4–5 minutes, turning occasionally, until crisp and golden.

- Drain on kitchen paper and serve with sweet chilli sauce for dipping.

 Spiced Chickpea Purée and Sweet Chilli Pittas Place a 400 g (13 oz) can chickpeas (rinsed and drained) in a saucepan with the juice and bring to the boil. Reduce the heat and simmer for 4 minutes until piping hot. Drain and transfer to a food processor with 1 tablespoon olive oil, ½ teaspoon each of ground cumin, ground coriander and paprika and 3 tablespoons chopped coriander. Squeeze in the juice of 1 lemon and whizz until smooth. Lightly toast 4 mini pitta breads, then split and fill with the purée along with a handful of spinach leaves and a drizzle of sweet chilli sauce.

Spicy Chickpea Cakes with Sweet Chilli Sauce Whizz a 400 g (13 oz) can chickpeas, drained and rinsed, in a food processor with 1 teaspoon minced garlic, ½ teaspoon each of ground cumin, coriander and paprika, ¼ teaspoon turmeric, 75 g (3 oz) wholemeal breadcrumbs and 1 egg yolk. Divide into 4 patties. Heat 3 tablespoons vegetable oil in a large heavy-based frying pan and cook the patties for 2 minutes on each side. Serve with sweet chilli sauce.

KID-FORA-VII

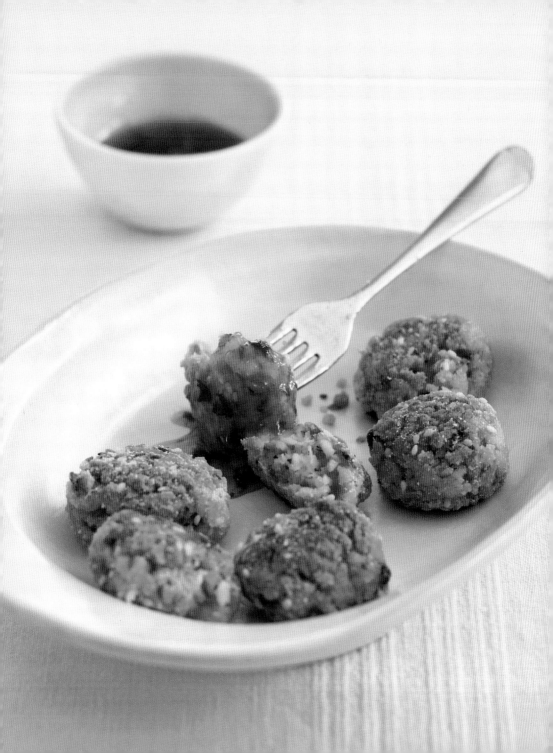

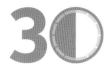

Chilli and Mustard Turkey Meatballs and Herb Tomato Sauce

Serves 4

375 g (12 oz) minced turkey
4 tablespoons chopped parsley
½ classic red chilli, deseeded and
finely chopped
1 tablespoon wholegrain mustard
plain flour, for dusting
3 tablespoons olive oil
500 ml (17 fl oz) passata
4 tablespoons chopped basil
200 g (7 oz) spaghetti
grated Parmesan cheese, to serve
(optional)

- Place the mince in a food processor with the parsley, chilli and mustard and whizz until well blended. Remove from the bowl and, using well-floured hands, shape the mixture into about 12–16 small walnut-sized balls.

- Heat the oil in a large heavy-based frying pan and cook the meatballs over a medium heat for 10–15 minutes, turning frequently, until the balls are golden and cooked through. Add the passata and basil and cook for a further 5 minutes until piping hot.

- Cook the spaghetti in a large saucepan of lightly salted boiling water for 8–10 minutes until tender. Drain and keep warm.

- Serve the meatballs and tomato sauce on top of the spaghetti in warmed serving bowls. Sprinkle with Parmesan, if liked.

Chillied Turkey Strips in a Tomato and Mustard Sauce Slice 375 g (12 oz) turkey steaks into thin strips. Heat 3 tablespoons vegetable oil in a large frying pan and cook the turkey for 5 minutes until golden, stirring occasionally. Add 1 teaspoon mild chilli powder and stir to coat. Add 300 ml (½ pint) passata and some pepper and bring to the boil. Cover and simmer for 3 minutes. Add 1 tablespoon wholegrain mustard and 1 tablespoon chopped parsley and serve with rice or mash.

Chilli and Mustard Turkey Burgers and Homemade Tomato Sauce Place 375 g (12 oz) minced turkey in a food processor with 4 tablespoons chopped parsley, ½ deseeded and finely chopped classic red chilli and 1 tablespoon wholegrain mustard and whizz until well blended. Divide the mixture into 4 pieces, then shape into patties. Heat 1 tablespoon olive oil in a large heavy-based nonstick frying pan and cook the burgers over a medium heat for 3–4 minutes on each side until golden and cooked through.

Meanwhile, make the tomato sauce. Place 150 ml (¼ pint) passata in a small saucepan with 1 tablespoon red wine vinegar, 2 tablespoons soft light brown sugar and ½ teaspoon paprika. Begin to heat, stirring continually, increasing the heat but taking care the passata does not spit while cooking, until the sugar has melted and the sauce is smooth. Transfer to a small serving bowl. Put the burgers into cut wholemeal soft round buns, spoon over the tomato sauce and serve with salad.

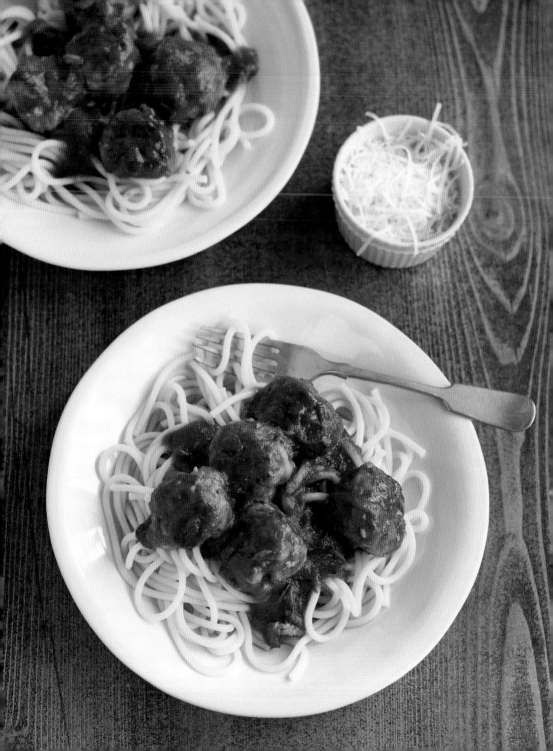

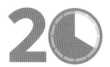

Gnocchi Pasta Gratin

Serves 4

500 g (1 lb) pack gnocchi

2 tablespoons olive oil

350 ml (12 fl oz) ready-made arrabbiata tomato sauce

4 tablespoons sunblush tomato paste

125 g (4 oz) pitted black olives, drained

150 g (5 oz) mozzarella cheese, drained and thinly sliced

4 tablespoons grated pecorino cheese

pepper

basil leaves, to garnish

To serve

garlic bread (optional)

salad (optional)

- Cook the gnocchi in a large saucepan of lightly salted boiling water, for 3–4 minutes or according to the packet instructions, then drain. Toss with the oil and season with pepper.

- Meanwhile, place the arrabbiata sauce and sunblush tomato paste in a saucepan and heat for 2 minutes until hot. Toss the gnocchi into the sauce and add the olives. Toss well, then transfer to a shallow gratin dish and arrange the mozzarella slices on top. Scatter the grated pecorino over the top of the mozzarella, then cook under a preheated hot grill for 8–10 minutes until golden and bubbling.

- Serve hot, garnished with basil leaves, with garlic bread and salad, if liked.

Gnocchi with Cherry Tomato Sauce Cook the gnocchi in a large pan of lightly salted boiling water, for 3–4 minutes or according to the packet instructions, then drain and return to the pan. Add 1 tablespoon olive oil, and season with pepper. Add a 400 g (13 oz) can cherry tomatoes and 2 tablespoons sundried tomato paste and cook over a high heat for 5 minutes until piping hot and cooked through. Serve in warmed serving bowls with grated pecorino.

Creamy Gnocchi and Aubergine Bake Cook 350 g (11½ oz) gnocchi in a large saucepan of lightly salted boiling water for 3–4 minutes or according to the packet instructions. Meanwhile, heat 500 ml (17 fl oz) ready-made tomato pasta sauce for 2–3 minutes until piping hot. Drain the gnocchi well and toss with a 400 g (13 oz) jar antipasti peppers, drained, a 400 g (13 oz) jar aubergine antipasti and the hot tomato sauce. Transfer to a large gratin dish. Mix 300 ml (½ pint) natural yogurt with 2 eggs and 2 tablespoons grated Parmesan cheese. Pour over the top of the gnocchi and spread evenly to the edges. Sprinkle with 3 tablespoons grated Parmesan and bake in a preheated oven, 220°C (425°F), Gas Mark 7, for 20 minutes until golden and piping hot.

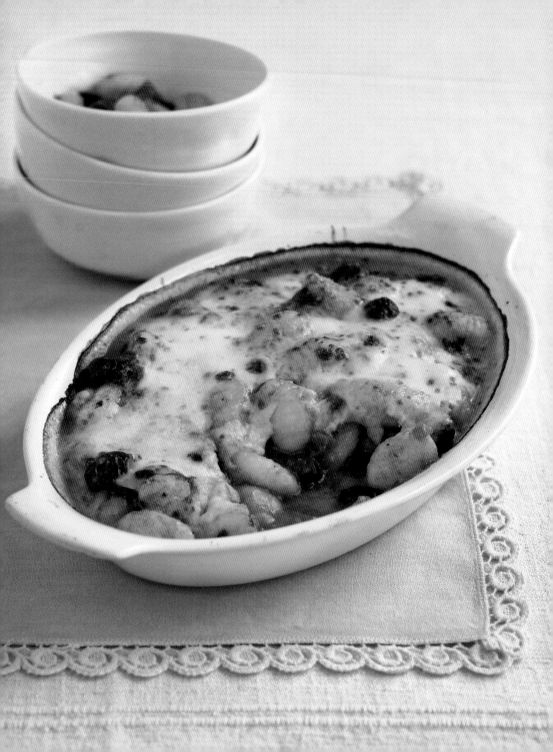

30 Tuna, Pepper and Cheese Calzones

Makes 4

1 x 145 g (5 oz) packets pizza
base mix
flour, for dusting
200 g (7 oz) can tuna, drained
1 small green pepper, cored,
deseeded and roughly chopped
50 g (2 oz) Cheddar cheese,
grated
salad, to serve (optional)

- Tip the pizza base mix into a bowl and make up with warm water according to the packet instructions. Divide into 4 pieces, place on a lightly floured surface and knead briefly to produce smooth balls of dough. Roll out each ball to about a 20 cm (8 inch) circle.

- Mix together the tuna, green pepper and cheese in a bowl, then divide the mixture between the 4 circles. Lightly brush the rims with a little cold water, then fold the dough over the filling and press to form a half-circle. Place the 4 half-circles on baking sheets and bake in a preheated oven, 220°C (425°F), Gas Mark 7, for 15–18 minutes until golden and cooked.

- Serve hot or warm with salad, if liked.

---

1 Tuna, Pepper and Cheese Wraps

Mix a 200 g (7 oz) can tuna, drained, with ½ cored, deseeded and thinly sliced green pepper and 1 tablespoon mayonnaise and season with pepper. Spread the tuna mayonnaise over the top of 2 flour tortillas, scatter each with 25 g (1 oz) grated Cheddar cheese and roll tightly to form a pinwheel effect. Cut each in half and serve with a handful of cherry tomato halves as a delicious dinner on the move.

2 Melted Tuna, Pepper and Cheese

Triangles Place a 200 g (7 oz) can tuna, drained, in a bowl with 1 small cored, deseeded and chopped green pepper, 1 small cored, deseeded and chopped red pepper and 50 g (2 oz) grated Cheddar cheese. Use to fill each of 4 flour tortillas in one quarter of the circle. Fold the wraps into 4 to enclose the filling, then place in a shallow flameproof dish. Arrange 150 g (5 oz) drained and thinly sliced mozzarella over the tortillas,

scatter over a further 25 g (1 oz) grated Cheddar cheese and cook under a preheated grill for 5 minutes until hot, bubbling and golden. Serve with a simple salad.

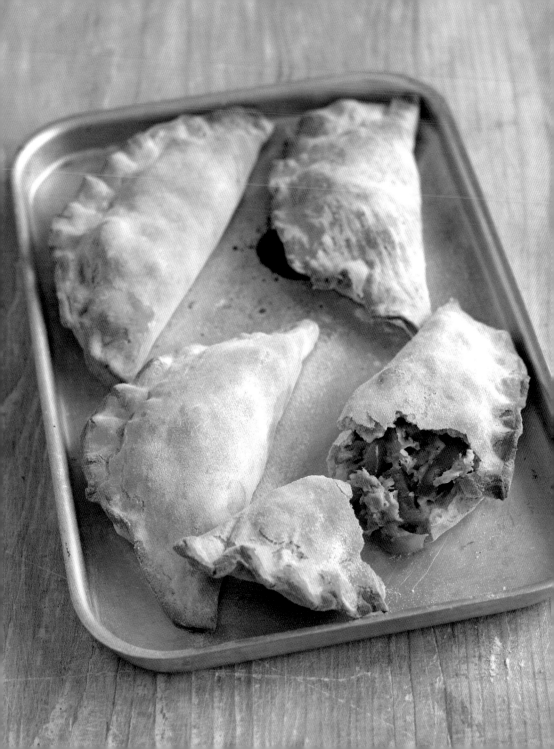

30 Scrambled Egg Enchiladas with Spinach and Tomatoes

Serves 4

3 tablespoons olive oil
1 small red onion, chopped
1 garlic clove, crushed
1 small red pepper, cored, deseeded and cut into strips
1 red chilli, cored, deseeded and chopped
½ teaspoon smoked paprika
pinch of ground coriander
25 g (1 oz) butter
4 eggs, beaten
4 soft flour tortillas
2 handfuls of baby spinach leaves
75 g (3 oz) Cheddar cheese, grated
2 tomatoes, chopped
salt and pepper

- Heat the oil in a small frying pan, add the onion, garlic, red pepper and chilli and cook over a low heat, stirring occasionally, for 10 minutes until very soft and tender. Stir in the paprika and coriander, season with salt and pepper and cook for a further 2 minutes.

- Melt the butter in a separate small saucepan (preferably nonstick). Season the eggs with salt and pepper and pour into the pan. Cook over a low heat, stirring, until the egg is softly set and scrambled, then remove from the heat.

- Lay the tortillas out on a board, arrange the spinach leaves on top, then spoon over the onion mixture and the scrambled egg. Fold the tortillas into triangles to enclose the filling and place in an ovenproof dish. Scatter the cheese and chopped tomatoes over the top and bake in a preheated oven, 200°C (400°F), Gas Mark 6, for 10 minutes until the cheese is melted and bubbling.

 Scrambled Egg and Tomato Burritos

Beat 4 eggs and season with salt and pepper, ½ teaspoon smoked paprika and a pinch of ground cumin. Melt 25 g (1 oz) butter in a nonstick saucepan, add the eggs and stir over a low heat until softly scrambled. Spoon on to warmed soft flour tortillas with a spoonful of ready-made tomato salsa and a handful of baby spinach leaves. Roll up to enclose the filling and serve.

 Mexican Baked Eggs

Heat 3 tablespoons olive oil in a frying pan and fry 1 chopped red onion, 1 crushed garlic clove, 2 cored, deseeded and sliced red peppers and 1 deseeded and chopped red pepper for 5 minutes to soften. Stir in ½ teaspoon smoked paprika, a pinch of ground cumin and 2 chopped tomatoes. Season with salt and pepper and cook for 5 minutes, stirring occasionally.

Transfer to an ovenproof dish and make 4 dips in the mixture. Break an egg into each dip and sprinkle over 50 g (2 oz) grated Cheddar cheese. Bake in a preheated oven, 200°C (400°F), Gas Mark 6, for 10 minutes until the egg whites are set and the yolks still soft. Serve with warmed tortillas.

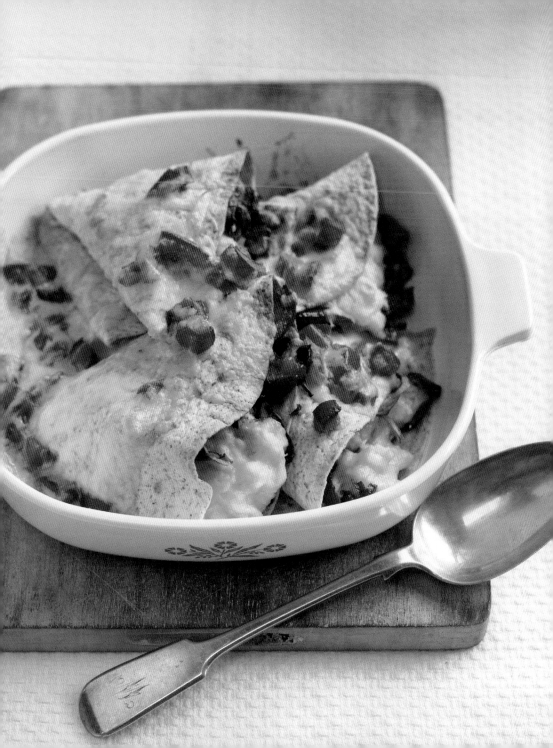

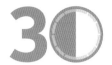

Beef Meatballs with Gravy and Baked Fries

Serves 4

2 baking potatoes, about 250 g (8 oz) each, scrubbed
3 tablespoons sunflower oil
500 g (1 lb) lean minced beef
½ onion, finely chopped
1 garlic clove, crushed
1 egg yolk
1 tablespoon plain flour, plus extra for coating
300 ml (½ pint) rich beef stock
1 tablespoon tomato purée
salt and pepper
broccoli, to serve

- Cut the potatoes into chip-sized pieces and toss in 2 tablespoons of the oil. Spread over a baking sheet in a single layer and season with salt and pepper. Bake in a preheated oven, 220°C (425°F), Gas Mark 7, for 25 minutes, turning occasionally, until golden and cooked through.

- Meanwhile, place the mince in a bowl with the onion, garlic and egg yolk. Season with salt and pepper and mix well. Roll the mixture into 12 even-sized balls and roll in flour to coat. Heat the remaining oil in a large frying pan, add the meatballs and fry over a medium heat for 10 minutes, turning occasionally, until browned and cooked through. Remove from the pan and set aside.

- Add the flour to the pan and cook, stirring, for 1 minute. Pour in the stock, bring to the boil, stir in the tomato purée and simmer for 2 minutes. Remove from the heat and return the meatballs to the pan and heat through. Serve with the veg.

 Spicy Tomato Meatballs with Couscous Place 250 g (8 oz) couscous in a heatproof bowl and add enough boiling water to cover by 1 cm (½ inch). Cover with clingfilm and leave for 5 minutes. Put 350 g (11½ oz) cooked Swedish-style meatballs into a pan, add 350 g (11½ oz) ready-made tomato pasta sauce and a pinch of chilli powder and heat for 5 minutes. Add a knob of butter to the couscous, season and fluff up with a fork until the butter has melted. Serve with the meatballs and tomato sauce.

 Creamy Meatball Pasta Cook 375 g (12 oz) penne or rigatoni in a large saucepan of lightly salted boiling water for 10 minutes until just tender. Meanwhile, heat 2 tablespoons sunflower oil in a large frying pan, add 350 g (11½ oz) ready-made beef meatballs and fry for 5 minutes until browned and cooked through. Remove from the pan and set aside. Add 125 g (4 oz) sliced mushrooms and 1 chopped courgette to the pan and fry for 2 minutes. Stir in 4 tablespoons crème fraîche and heat through, adding a little water if the sauce is too thick. Return the meatballs to the pan and heat through. Drain the pasta, add to the pan and mix well. Add 2 tablespoons chopped parsley and sprinkle with grated cheese to serve.

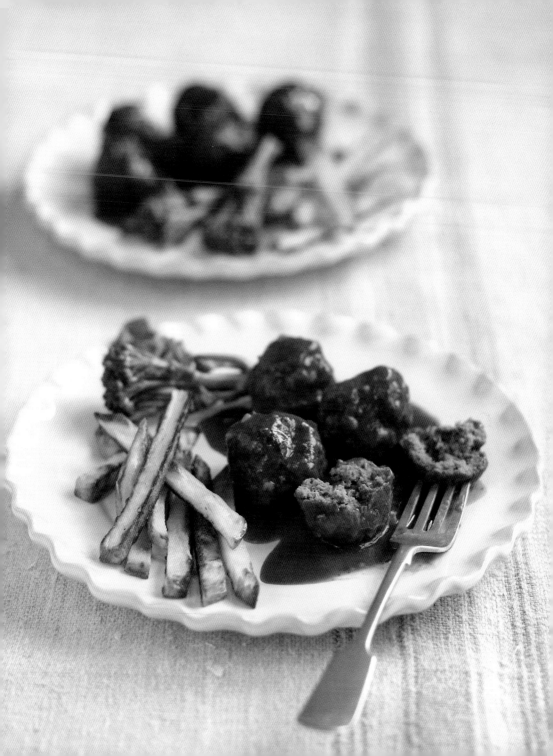

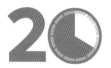 # Salmon and Broccoli Fishcakes

Makes 4

75 g (3 oz) broccoli florets
40 g (1½ oz) instant mashed
  potato
1 tablespoon grated Parmesan
  cheese
250 g (8 oz) salmon fillet
4 tablespoons plain flour, plus
  extra for dusting
1 egg, beaten
150 g (5 oz) wholemeal
  breadcrumbs
5 tablespoons vegetable oil
mixed peas and sweetcorn, to
  serve (optional)

- Cook the broccoli florets in a saucepan of lightly salted boiling water for 3 minutes. Drain, rinse with cold water and chop into small pieces. Make up the mash according to the packet instructions, add the Parmesan and mix well.

- Place the salmon on a microwave-proof plate and cover with clingfilm. Cook for 2–3 minutes until the fish is opaque.

- Mix the potato with the broccoli and salmon, then divide into 4 pieces. Shape into patties, using metal spoons if the mixture is too hot to handle. Put the flour on one plate, the beaten egg on another and the breadcrumbs on a third. Lightly roll the fishcakes in the flour, then the egg and finally the breadcrumbs.

- Heat the oil in a large heavy-based frying pan and cook the fishcakes for 2–3 minutes on each side. Drain on kitchen paper and serve with peas and sweetcorn, if liked.

 Pan-Fried Salmon and Broccoli

Season 2 x 150 g (5 oz) salmon steaks with pepper. Heat 15 g (½ oz) butter in a frying pan and cook the steaks for 5–7 minutes, turning once, until golden. Meanwhile, heat 2 tablespoons olive oil in a frying pan and cook 175 g (6 oz) tenderstem broccoli, cut into small florets with some stem, for 5 minutes, turning occasionally and adding 2 tablespoons water for the final 2 minutes. Serve the salmon and broccoli with grated Parmesan cheese.

Salmon and Broccoli Pie

Cook 250 g (8 oz) broccoli florets in lightly salted boiling water for 5 minutes until just tender, then drain. Meanwhile, place 375 g (12 oz) salmon fillets in a frying pan with 150 ml (¼ pint) water and bring to the boil, cover tightly and simmer for 5 minutes until the fish is opaque. Reserve the cooking liquid. Heat 25 g (1 oz) butter in a saucepan until melted. Add 25 g (1 oz) flour and cook over a low heat for a few seconds. Remove from the heat and gradually add

300 ml (½ pint) milk, a little at a time, stirring well. Once all the milk is added, return to the heat and bring to the boil, stirring until thickened. Stir in the reserved cooking liquid and 4 tablespoons grated Parmesan cheese. Flake the salmon, add to the sauce with the broccoli and fold in. Transfer to a shallow gratin dish. Mix 750 g (1½ lb) chilled ready-made mashed potato to loosen. Spoon over the salmon, scatter with 3 tablespoons grated Parmesan. Cook under a preheated grill for 5–8 minutes until golden.

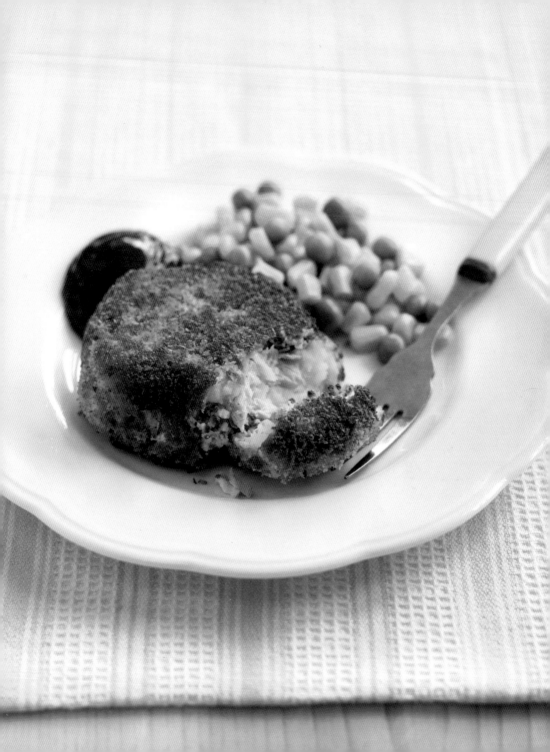

10 Creamy Pork and Peppers

Serves 4

2 tablespoons olive oil

375 g (12 oz) pork fillet or similar, cut into strips

1 tablespoon smoked paprika

300 g (10 oz) ready-made tomato pasta sauce

150 ml (¼ pint) soured cream

300 g (10 oz) antipasti peppers, drained

chopped parsley, to garnish

- Heat the oil in a large heavy-based frying pan and cook the pork over a high heat for 5 minutes until golden and cooked through.

- Add the paprika and cook for a few seconds, then add the pasta sauce and bring to the boil.

- Reduce the heat, add the soured cream and peppers and heat for 2–3 minutes until piping hot but not boiling.

- Scatter with chopped parsley to serve, if liked.

20 Creamy Pork Raxo

Heat 1 tablespoon olive oil in a large heavy-based frying pan and cook 1 small sliced red onion and 3 thinly sliced pork loin steaks, about 150 g (5 oz) each, for 5 minutes until golden. Add 2 teaspoons smoked paprika and ½ teaspoon ground cumin and cook for 1 minute, then add 2 tablespoons sun-dried tomato paste and 200 g (7 oz) canned chopped tomatoes. Cook, stirring, for a further 2 minutes, then add 6 tablespoons water. Add 200 ml (7 fl oz) crème fraîche and cook and stir for 2 minutes more until piping hot. Serve with rice or chips.

30 Pork and Pepper Goulash

Heat 1 tablespoon olive oil in a large heavy-based saucepan and cook 1 large red onion, 1 cored, deseeded and chopped green pepper, 1 cored, deseeded and chopped red pepper and 4 x 150 g (5 oz) thinly sliced pork loin steaks over a high heat for 8–10 minutes until the pork is golden. Add 1 tablespoon smoked paprika and 1 teaspoon ground cumin and cook for 1 minute, then add a 400 g (13 oz) can chopped tomatoes, 450 ml (¾ pint) chicken stock and 1 tablespoon sun-dried tomato paste and bring to the boil. Cover and simmer for 15 minutes. Serve ladled over hot rice with spoonfuls of soured cream and garnished with parsley, if liked.

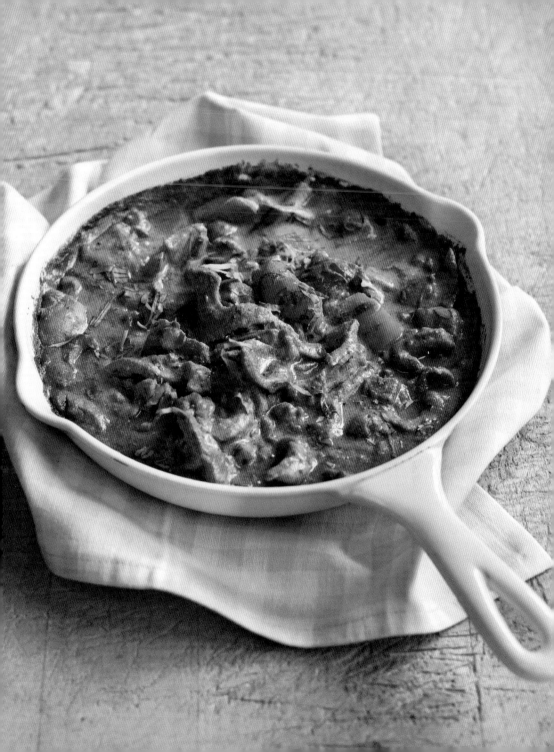

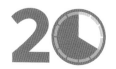

Lemon Cod Goujons with 'Caperless' Tartare Sauce

Serves 4

about 600 ml (1 pint) vegetable oil

500 g (1 lb) cod loin, cut into chunky pieces

125 g (4 oz) plain flour

1 teaspoon paprika

2 eggs, beaten

250 g (8 oz) breadcrumbs

3 tablespoons chopped parsley

grated rind of 1 lemon

pepper

peas, to serve (optional)

For the tartare sauce

3 tablespoons mayonnaise

3 tablespoons crème fraîche

½ teaspoon Dijon mustard

1 gherkin, finely chopped

1 tablespoon chopped parsley

- Pour the vegetable oil into a medium-sized deep saucepan and begin to heat ready to fry the goujons.

- Meanwhile, place the cod pieces in a bowl, add the flour and paprika and season with pepper. Toss well to lightly coat the fish. Place the beaten eggs in one bowl and the breadcrumbs, parsley and lemon rind in another. Toss the fish pieces in the egg, then in the lemon and herb breadcrumbs, pressing firmly to coat.

- Test the oil to see if it is hot enough – lower a small piece of bread into the oil and if it turns brown in 20 seconds the oil is ready. Carefully lower the fish pieces into the hot oil and cook for 3–4 minutes until golden and cooked through. Remove from the oil using a slotted spoon and drain on kitchen paper.

- To make the tartare sauce, mix the mayonnaise with the crème fraîche and mustard, then fold in the chopped gherkin and parsley.

- Serve the goujons with the sauce to dip and peas, if liked.

 Lemon and Pepper Cod Cubes with Herby Mayonnaise Put 375 g (12 oz) cubed cod loin in a bowl with 3 tablespoons plain flour, ½ teaspoon paprika and the grated rind of 1 lemon. Toss well. Heat 6 tablespoons olive oil in a large heavy-based frying pan. Cook the fish cubes for 5 minutes, turning occasionally. Meanwhile, mix 5 tablespoons mayonnaise with 1 tablespoon chopped herbs and serve with the fish.

 Lemony Roasted Cod Loin with 'Caperless' Tartare Sauce Place 4 pieces of cod loin (about 125 g/4 oz each) in a lightly oiled large roasting tin. Mix 250 g (8 oz) halved baby new potatoes and 375 g (12 oz) peeled and chunky cut carrots with 1 tablespoon olive oil and scatter around the fish. Scatter over 3 tablespoons chopped parsley and the grated rind of 1 lemon and bake in a preheated oven, 200°C (400°F), Gas Mark 6, for 20 minutes until the vegetables are tender and the fish is opaque and cooked through. Meanwhile, make the tartare sauce as above and serve with the fish and vegetables.

KID-FORA-LUI

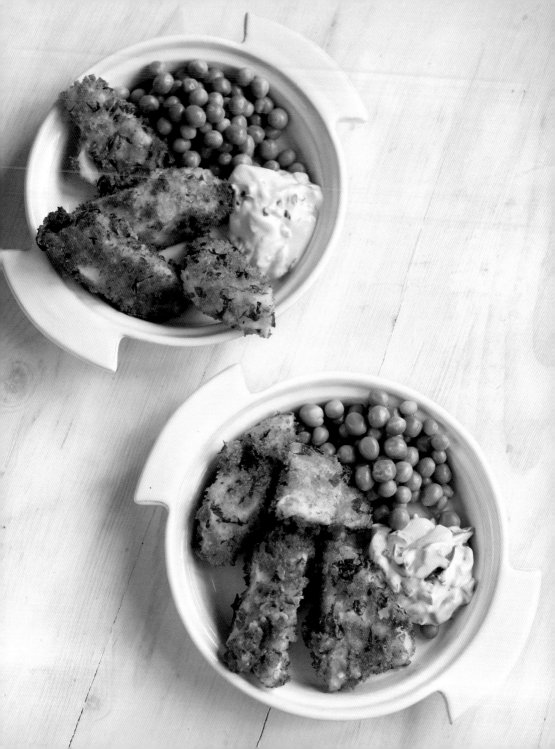

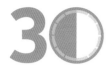 # Chicken, Bacon and Leek Pies

Serves 4

150 g (5 oz) ready-rolled
   shortcrust pastry
beaten egg, to glaze
1 tablespoon olive oil
40 g (1½ oz) butter
375 g (12 oz) chicken breast, cut
   into small chunks
8 back bacon rashers, cut into
   pieces
2 leeks, rinsed, trimmed and cut
   into slices
25 g (1 oz) plain flour
300 ml (½ pint) milk
1 teaspoon Dijon mustard
200 ml (7 fl oz) crème fraîche
salt and pepper
green vegetables, to serve

- Line a baking sheet with greaseproof paper. Cut the pastry into 4 equal rectangles or squares and place on the baking sheet so the pastry is not lying completely flat, lightly brush with beaten egg and bake in a preheated oven, 200 °C (400 °F), Gas Mark 6, for 12–15 minutes until golden.

- Meanwhile, heat the oil and 15 g (½ oz) of the butter in a heavy-based frying pan and cook the chicken and bacon over a high heat for 8–10 minutes until golden. Add the leeks and cook for 5 minutes. Remove from the heat and set aside.

- Heat the remaining butter in a saucepan and add the flour. Cook for a few seconds, remove from the heat and add the milk, a little at a time, stirring well after each addition. Add the mustard, return to the heat and bring to the boil, stirring, until boiled and thickened. Add the crème fraîche and cook for 1–2 minutes. Season, then pour into the pan with the chicken and stir. Ladle the chicken onto 4 serving plates, top each with a pastry rectangle and serve with green veg.

 Chicken, Bacon and Leek Sauté

Cut 2 x 175 g (6 oz) chicken breasts in half length-ways. Heat 25 g (1 oz) butter in a pan and cook the pieces over a medium heat for 5–6 minutes, turning once, until cooked. Heat 25 g (1 oz) butter in a frying pan and cook 3 roughly snipped bacon rashers and 2 roughly chopped leeks over a high heat for 5 minutes until soft. Add 200 ml (7 fl oz) crème fraîche and 1 teaspoon Dijon mustard and bring to the boil. Spoon the hot sauce over the chicken and serve.

 Chicken, Bacon and Leeks with Potato Cakes Heat 1 tablespoon olive oil and 15 g (½ oz) butter in a large heavy-based frying pan. Cook 375 g (12 oz) chicken breast, cut into small chunks, and 8 back bacon rashers, cut into pieces, for 8–10 minutes until golden. Add 2 leeks, rinsed, trimmed and cut into slices, and cook for a further 5 minutes until the leeks are tender and soft. Add 2 x 295 g (10 oz) cans condensed chicken soup and heat for 5 minutes until piping hot. Meanwhile, cook 4 ready-made potato cakes under a preheated hot grill for 2–3 minutes until lightly toasted on the top and piping hot. Ladle the chicken and bacon mixture on to warm serving plates and top each with a hot potato cake.

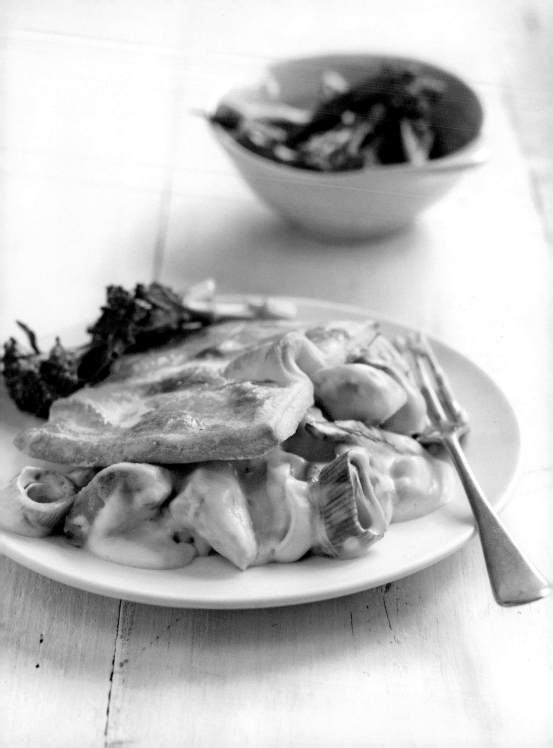

30 Chicken, Chorizo and Prawn Jambalaya

Serves 4

1 tablespoon olive oil

175 g (6 oz) chicken breast, thinly sliced

125 g (4 oz) chorizo, thinly sliced

1 red pepper, cored, deseeded and roughly chopped

1 teaspoon Cajun spice

200 g (7 oz) paella rice

400 g (13 oz) can chopped tomatoes

125 g (4 oz) okra, roughly chopped

900 ml (1½ pints) chicken stock

50 g (2 oz) raw peeled prawns

warm crusty bread, to serve

- Heat the oil in a large heavy-based frying pan and cook the chicken, chorizo and red pepper over a high heat for 5 minutes until golden.

- Add the Cajun spice and stir to coat, then add the rice, tomatoes and okra and stir again. Pour in the stock and bring to the boil, then reduce the heat, cover and simmer for 20–25 minutes, stirring occasionally, until the rice is tender, topping up with water if necessary.

- Add the prawns for the final 10 minutes of cooking and stir into the rice to heat through.

- Serve with warm crusty bread.

 10 Chicken, Chorizo and Tomato Stew

Heat 1 tablespoon olive oil in a nonstick saucepan and cook 250 g (8 oz) chicken breast, cut into small cubes, and 125 g (4 oz) thinly sliced chorizo over a high heat for 5 minutes. Add 1 teaspoon Cajun spice, 2 x 400 g (13 oz) cans chopped tomatoes and 125 g (4 oz) frozen peas. Bring to the boil, then simmer for 3 minutes until piping hot. Serve ladled over express rice or instant mashed potato.

 20 Chicken, Prawn and Chorizo Pilaff

Cook 175 g (6 oz) easy-cook long grain rice in a large saucepan of lightly salted boiling water for 12–15 minutes until tender, then drain. Meanwhile, heat 2 tablespoons olive oil in a large heavy-based frying pan and cook 250 g (8 oz) thinly sliced chicken breast, 125 g (4 oz) thinly sliced chorizo sausage and 1 cored, deseeded and roughly chopped red pepper over a high heat for 10 minutes until cooked and softened. Add 1 teaspoon Cajun spice and stir, then add 125 g (4 oz) frozen peas and cook for 2 minutes. Add the drained rice and stir-fry for 3–4 minutes until all the ingredients are piping hot and cooked through.

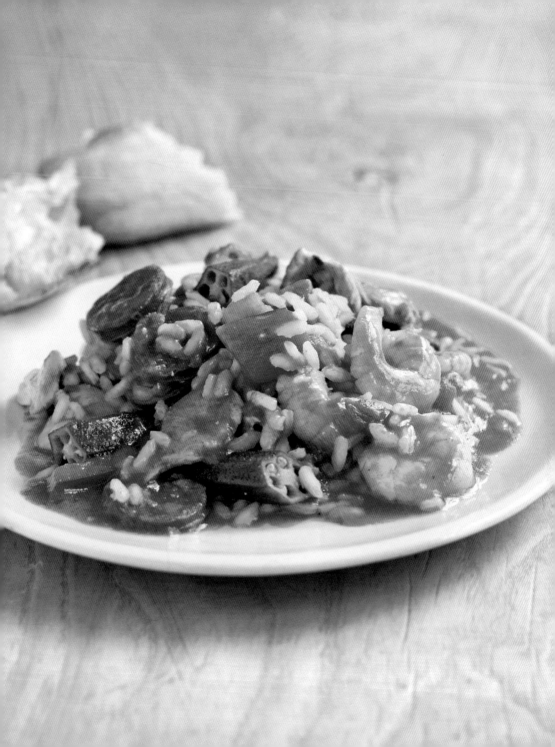

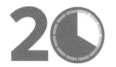

Pork Dumplings with Dipping Sauce

Serves 4

200 g (7 oz) minced pork
2 spring onions, roughly chopped
4 canned water chestnuts, roughly chopped
½ teaspoon ginger purée from a jar or tube
1 tablespoon soy sauce
1 tablespoon teriyaki sauce
24 wonton wrappers
1 tablespoon sunflower oil
125 ml (4 fl oz) water

For the dipping sauce

3 tablespoons soy sauce
2 tablespoons sweet chilli sauce
1 teaspoon sesame oil
juice of ½ lime

- Place the pork, spring onions, water chestnuts, ginger purée, soy sauce and teriyaki sauce in a food processor and pulse to make a rough paste. Place spoonfuls of the mixture in the centre of each wonton wrapper and lightly brush the edges with water. Gather up the edges to make a pasty shape and pleat the edges a few times to enclose the filling.

- Heat a large nonstick frying pan until hot. Add the oil and arrange the dumplings in a single layer in the pan (you may have to do this in 2 batches). Fry for 2 minutes, until golden on the bottom, then pour in the measurement water. Cover and cook for 6–7 minutes until the water has been absorbed.

- Mix together the dipping sauce ingredients and serve with the dumplings.

Sticky Pork Mini Wraps

Heat a nonstick frying pan or wok until very hot. Add 375 g (12 oz) minced pork and stir-fry for 5 minutes until browned and clumpy. Add 2 tablespoons teriyaki sauce and 1 tablespoon sweet chilli sauce and continue to cook until the mixture turns sticky. Serve in warmed pancakes (the sort you would use for crispy duck) with sticks of cucumber and extra teriyaki sauce for dipping.

Steamed Pork Dumplings with Chinese Vegetables

Blend 200 g (7 oz) minced pork with 2 chopped spring onions, 4 chopped canned water chestnuts, ½ teaspoon ginger purée, 1 tablespoon soy sauce and 1 tablespoon teriyaki sauce in a food processor. Place spoonfuls on 24 wonton wrappers and brush the edges with water. Gather the edges in the middle and scrunch to make purses. Lightly grease 2 bamboo steamer trays and arrange the dumplings in a single layer. Cover and steam for 5–6 minutes. Meanwhile, heat 1 tablespoon sunflower oil in a large wok or frying pan, add 250 g (8 oz) broccoli, cut into florets, 125 g (4 oz) mangetout and 1 head of pak choi, separated into leaves, and stir-fry for 3 minutes. Add 2 tablespoons sweet chilli sauce, 1 tablespoon soy sauce and 1 tablespoon teriyaki sauce. Bring to the boil, heat through and serve with the dumplings.

KID-FORA-GEM

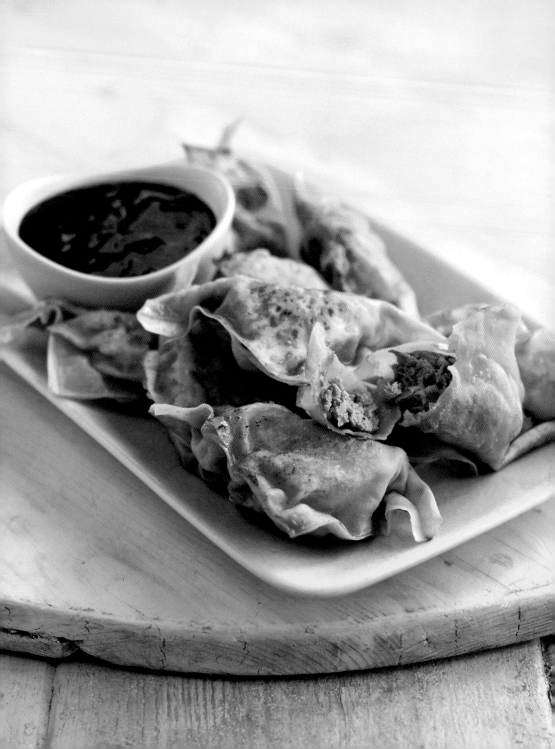

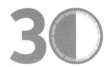

Creamy Pesto Fish Pie

Serves 4

500 g (1 lb) skinless white fish
  fillet, cut into chunks
3 tablespoons pesto
200 g (7 oz) crème fraîche
375 g (12 oz) ready-rolled puff
  pastry
beaten egg, to glaze
salt and pepper

To serve

new potatoes
green beans

- Scatter the chunks of fish evenly over the base of a shallow ovenproof dish. Stir the pesto into the crème fraîche in a bowl, then spoon over the fish. Season with salt and pepper.

- Unroll the pastry, place it over the dish to cover and trim off any excess with a sharp knife. Brush the pastry with beaten egg.

- Bake in a preheated oven, 200°C (400°F), Gas Mark 6, for 20–25 minutes until the pastry is risen and golden and the fish is cooked. Serve with new potatoes and green beans.

 Creamy Pesto Smoked Mackerel Tagliatelle Cook 500 g (1 lb) tagliatelle in a saucepan of lightly salted boiling water for 3 minutes until just cooked, then drain and tip back into the pan. Add 200 g (7 oz) crème fraîche, 1 tablespoon pesto, 150 g (5 oz) flaked smoked mackerel fillets, the juice of ½ lemon and 2 handfuls of baby spinach leaves. Heat, stirring gently, until the sauce comes to the boil. Season with salt and pepper and serve.

 Grilled Creamy Pesto Fish with Rosti Cakes Cook 8 small or 4 large frozen ready-made rosti cakes in the oven according to the packet instructions. Meanwhile, place 4 halved tomatoes on a baking sheet and sprinkle with a little grated Parmesan cheese. Bake in the oven. Place 4 pieces of skinless white fish fillet, about 150 g (5 oz) each, on a foil-lined grill pan that has been lightly oiled. Mix together 4 teaspoons pesto and 3 tablespoons crème fraîche in a bowl, then spoon over each piece of fish. Drizzle with a little olive oil and cook under a preheated medium grill for 8–10 minutes until the fish is cooked and opaque. Serve with the rosti cakes and baked tomatoes.

KID-FORA-NAM

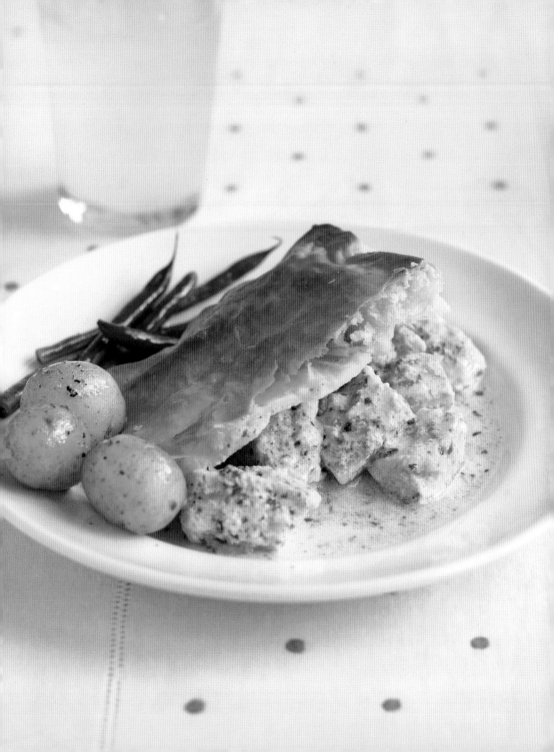

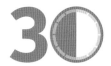

30 Sticky Chicken Drumsticks with Cucumber and Sweetcorn

Serves 4

8 small chicken drumsticks

4 tablespoons maple syrup

2 tablespoons soy sauce

2 tablespoons sesame oil

½ teaspoon Chinese five spice powder

¼ cucumber, thinly sliced

125 g (4 oz) canned sweetcorn, drained

1 red pepper, cored, deseeded and thinly sliced

3 tablespoons ready-made French dressing

pepper

• Make 3 deep slashes in the flesh of each of the chicken pieces. Mix together the maple syrup, soy sauce, sesame oil and Chinese five spice powder in a large mixing bowl, add the chicken thighs and toss to coat. Transfer to a roasting tin and pour over any of the remaining marinade. Roast in a preheated oven, 200°C (400°F), Gas Mark 6, for 25 minutes until the chicken is golden and cooked through.

• Meanwhile, make the salad. Place the cucumber, sweetcorn and red pepper in a bowl and toss well.

• Add the French dressing and toss well again, seasoning with pepper. Serve with the hot chicken.

---

1 Chicken Drumsticks with Sticky Dipping Sauce and Crudités Place 4 ready-cooked chicken drumsticks on a microwave-proof plate. Mix 3 tablespoons maple syrup with 2 tablespoons soy sauce and ½ teaspoon Chinese five spice powder. Brush liberally over the chicken, then heat for 8 minutes until piping hot. Meanwhile, cut 1 cored and deseeded red pepper and ½ cucumber into sticks and place on a serving platter. Mix 4 tablespoons hoi sin sauce with 1 tablespoon maple syrup and place in a bowl in the centre of the platter. Serve with the hot drumsticks for dipping.

2 Sticky Chicken and Vegetable Pan-Fry Heat 3 tablespoons sesame oil in a frying pan and cook 350 g (11½) thinly sliced chicken breast over a high heat for 3 minutes, then add 1 thinly sliced courgette and 1 cored, deseeded and sliced red pepper and fry for a further 5–6 minutes until golden and tender. Meanwhile, mix 3 tablespoons soy sauce with 3 tablespoons honey and ½ teaspoon Chinese five spice powder. Pour into the chicken and continue to cook over a high heat for 1 minute. Add 175 g (6 oz) canned sweetcorn, drained, and toss and cook for a further 5 minutes until piping hot. Serve with express rice, if liked.

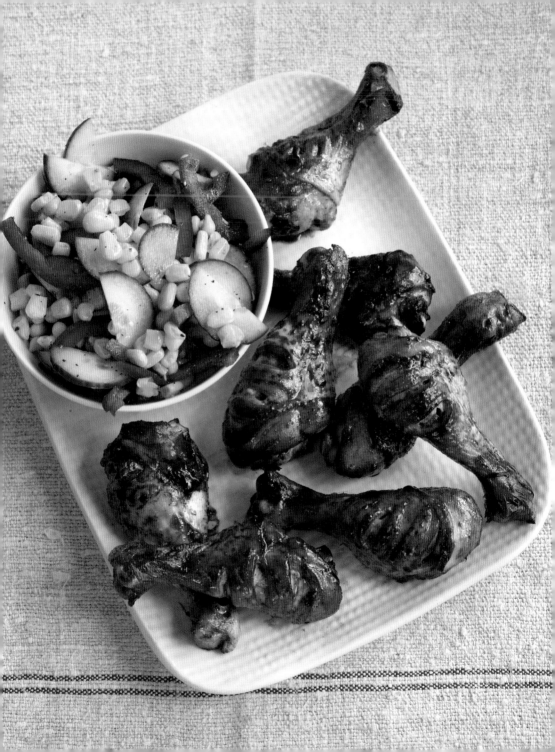

10 Curried Lamb Steak Sandwiches

Serves 4

2 lamb steaks, about 125 g
  (4 oz) each
1 teaspoon mild curry powder
2 tablespoons olive oil
4 thick slices of freshly cut
  wholemeal bread
2 tablespoons mango chutney
handful of salad leaves
pepper

- Place the lamb steaks between 2 sheets of clingfilm on a board and bash with a rolling pin until half thickness. Remove the clingfilm and season each side with a little pepper, then sprinkle each side with the curry powder to lightly coat.

- Heat the oil in a large frying pan and cook the steaks over a high heat for 3–4 minutes on each side until cooked through.

- Place the bread slices on a board and top each of 2 slices with 1 tablespoon mango chutney, then top with the hot lamb steak. Scatter with the salad leaves, and top each with another slice of bread.

- Cut each sandwich in half diagonally and serve 1 half per child.

2 Curried Lamb Burgers

Place 375 g (12 oz) minced lamb in a mixing bowl and season with pepper. Add 1 tablespoon mild curry powder and 3 tablespoons chopped coriander and mix well using a fork to mash the flavours together. Using your hands, divide the mixture into 4, then shape each piece into a burger. Place on a foil-lined grill rack and lightly brush with oil. Cook under a preheated grill for 3–4 minutes on each side until cooked through. Divide between 4 split wholemeal rolls and top with 1 tablespoon mango chutney and some salad leaves. Serve hot with halved cherry tomatoes.

3 Curried Lamb with Naan

Heat a large frying pan and cook 500 g (1 lb) minced lamb and 1 roughly chopped onion over a high heat for 10 minutes until browned. Add 2 tablespoons mild curry powder and cook for a further minute then add 300 ml (½ pint) lamb stock and a 400 g (13 oz) can chopped tomatoes. Bring to the boil, then reduce the heat, cover and simmer for 15 minutes until the lamb is cooked. Stir through 3 tablespoons chopped coriander. Warm 2 naan breads in a microwave or hot oven and serve the lamb ladled on to halves of warm naan.

KID-FORA-CUZ

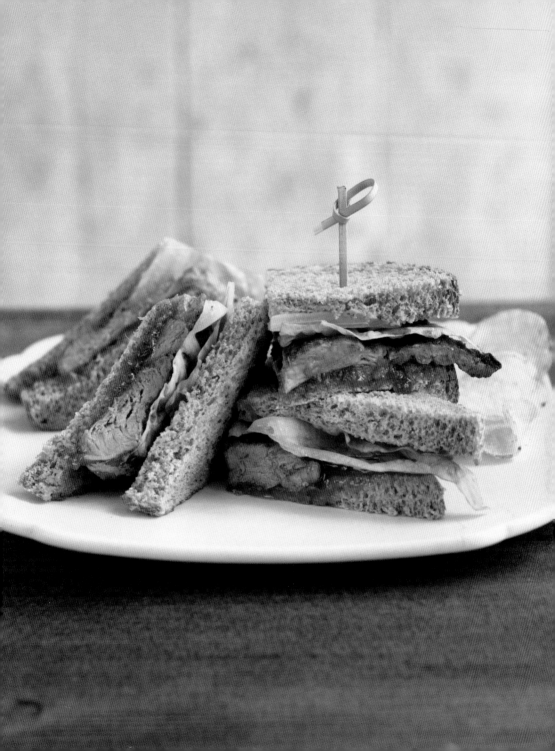

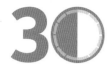

Sticky Pork Ribs with Homemade Baked Beans

Serves 4

1.25 kg (2½ lb) pork spare ribs
4 tablespoons runny honey
2 tablespoons soy sauce
2 garlic cloves, crushed
2 tablespoons tomato ketchup
crusty bread, to serve

For the beans

1 tablespoon sunflower oil
1 carrot, peeled and chopped
1 celery stick, chopped
400 g (13 oz) can haricot beans, rinsed and drained
400 g (13 oz) can chopped tomatoes
1 teaspoon paprika
1 teaspoon Worcestershire sauce
pinch of caster sugar

- Place the pork ribs in a large saucepan and cover with boiling water from the kettle. Cover and simmer for 10 minutes.

- In a small saucepan, gently melt the honey with the soy sauce, garlic and ketchup. Drain the ribs, place on a foil-lined baking sheet and pour over the honey mixture. Turn to coat evenly, then cook in a preheated oven, 220°C (425°F), Gas Mark 7, for 15 minutes, turning occasionally, until sticky and beginning to char at the edges.

- Meanwhile, make the beans. Heat the oil in a pan, add the carrot and celery and cook, stirring, for 5 minutes to soften. Add the beans, tomatoes, paprika, Worcestershire sauce and sugar, stir well and bring to a simmer. Cover and simmer gently for 15 minutes, stirring occasionally.

- Serve the ribs with the beans and crusty bread.

 Sausage and Smoky Bean Baguettes

Grill or fry 4 pork sausages until cooked through. Heat a 415 g (14 oz) can baked beans with ½ teaspoon smoked paprika and a dash of Worcestershire sauce in a saucepan. Cut 1 baguette into 4 pieces and split each piece almost in half lengthways. Butter the bread and fill each piece with a sausage and the baked beans.

 Maple Glazed Pork with Chilli Beans

Brush 8 streaky pork slices, about 75 g (3 oz) each, with maple syrup. Cook under a preheated medium grill for 8–10 minutes, turning occasionally, until golden, cooked through and starting to char at the edges. Meanwhile, heat 1 tablespoon sunflower oil in a frying pan, and fry 1 chopped onion and 1 deseeded and chopped green pepper cook for 5 minutes to soften. Add a 400 g (13 oz) can chopped tomatoes and 1 teaspoon mild chilli powder. Bring to the boil, add a 400 g (13 oz) can red kidney beans, drained and rinsed, cover and simmer for 10 minutes. Season with salt and pepper and serve with the maple pork slices and a dollop of soured cream.

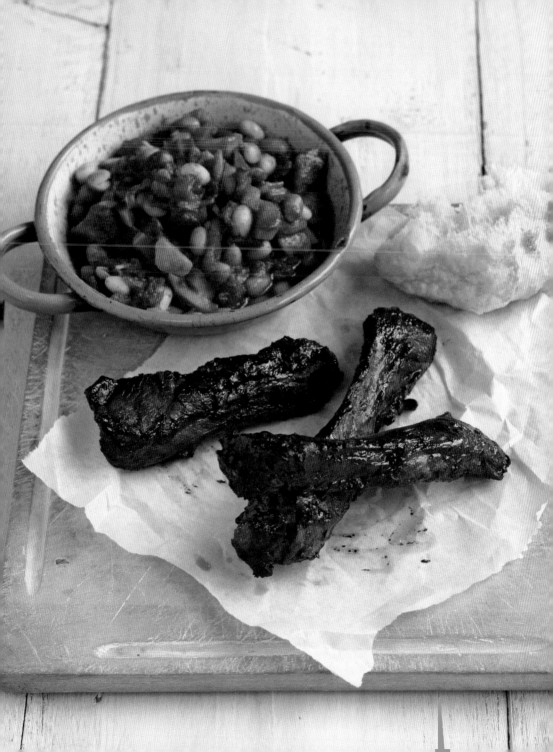

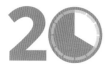

20 Crispy Chicken with Egg Fried Rice

Serves 4

sunflower oil, for deep frying
75 g (3 oz) plain flour
1 tablespoon cornflour
200 ml (7 fl oz) sparkling mineral
water
3 boneless, skinless chicken
breasts, cut into small chunks

For the fried rice

2 tablespoons sunflower oil
2 bacon rashers, chopped
4 spring onions, halved and cut
into thin strips
75 g (3 oz) mushrooms, sliced
200 g (7 oz) can sweetcorn,
75 g (3 oz) frozen peas
200 g (7 oz) ready-cooked rice
1 teaspoon Chinese five spice
1 tablespoon soy sauce
2 eggs, beaten

- Half-fill a wok or deep pan with sunflower oil and heat to 180–190°C (350–375°F) or until a cube of bread browns in 30 seconds. Meanwhile, mix together the flour, cornflour and a pinch of salt in a bowl. Pour in the sparkling water and mix using a hand whisk. Don't overmix – there should still be a few lumps.

- Quickly dip the chicken pieces into the batter, drain off the excess, then add to the hot oil about 6 pieces at a time. Fry for about 2 minutes until crisp and golden and the chicken is cooked. Remove with a slotted spoon, drain on kitchen paper and keep warm while cooking the remaining chicken.

- To make the fried rice, heat the oil in a large frying pan, add the bacon and fry for 3 minutes until crisp. Add the spring onions, the mushrooms, sweetcorn and peas and stir-fry for 2 minutes. Add the rice, Chinese five spice powder and soy sauce and heat through for 3 minutes until the rice is hot. Pour in the beaten eggs and stir until cooked.

- Serve the rice with the crispy chicken.

10 Sweet and Sour Chicken and Rice

Stir-Fry Heat 1 tablespoon sunflower oil in a wok and stir-fry 250 g thinly sliced chicken breast with 2 chopped bacon rashers for 3 minutes. Add 200 g (7 oz) frozen mixed vegetables and 400 g (13 oz) frozen ready-cooked rice. Stir in 125 g (4 oz) sweet and sour stir-fry sauce and 1 tablespoon soy sauce and heat through.

30 Crispy Sweet and Sour Chicken

Mix 75 g (3 oz) plain flour, 1 tablespoon cornflour and 200 ml (7 fl oz) sparking mineral water to make a lumpy batter. Cut 3 boneless, skinless chicken breasts, into chunks, dip into the batter, drain off excess, then deep-fry, in batches, in a pan half-filled with sunflower oil heated to 180°C (350°F). Fry for 2 minutes until golden, crisp and cooked. Drain on kitchen paper. Heat 1 tablespoon sunflower oil in a wok and stir-fry 1 chopped onion, 1 carrot, thinly sliced, 1 red pepper, deseeded and thinly sliced, and 75 g (3 oz) baby corn, for 2 minutes. Add 225 g (7½ oz) canned pineapple chunks (drained, juice reserved). Heat through. Mix a little of the pineapple juice with 2 tablespoons cornflour to make a smooth paste. Add the remaining juice, 2 tablespoons tomato sauce, 2 tablespoons vinegar and 1 tablespoon soft brown sugar to the pan and bring to the boil, stirring, to thicken. Stir in the chicken and serve with rice.

KID-FORA-KIO

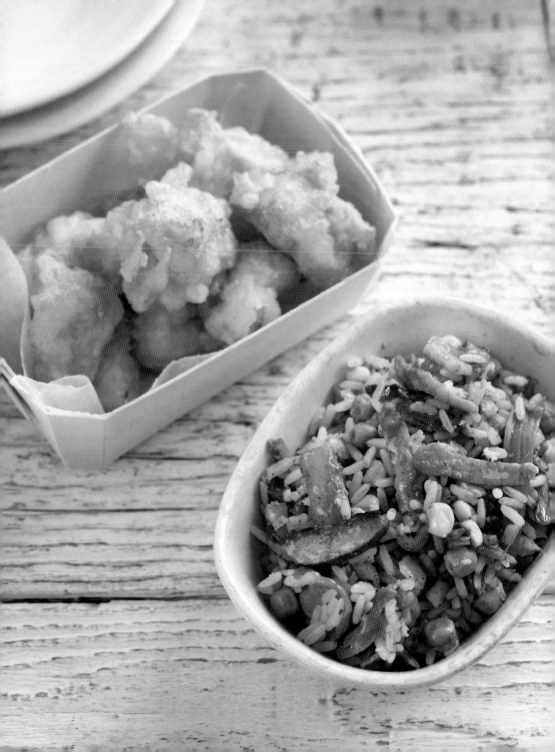

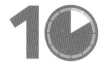

Sausage, Tomato and Pepper Pan-Fry

Serves 4

1 tablespoon olive oil
24 baby cocktail sausages,
 wrapped in bacon
1 thinly sliced red pepper
1 thinly sliced yellow pepper
½ teaspoon smoked paprika
400 g (13 fl oz) can chopped
 tomatoes with herbs
cooked wholemeal rice or
 ready-made mash, to serve

- Heat the oil in a large heavy-based frying pan and cook the sausages over a medium-high heat for 2–3 minutes until beginning to turn golden. Add the peppers and cook for a further 3 minutes, stirring occasionally, until softened.

- Add the smoked paprika and stir well, then add the tomatoes and cook for a further 2 minutes until piping hot and the sausages are cooked through.

- Serve hot ladled on to wholemeal rice or ready-made mash.

---

2 **Smoky Sausage, Tomato and Pepper Casserole** Cook 12 chipolata sausages under a preheated hot grill for 10–12 minutes, turning. Heat 2 tablespoons olive oil in a heavy-based frying pan and cook 1 chopped onion for 2 minutes. Add 1 orange and 1 red sliced pepper and cook for 3 minutes. Add 1 tablespoon smoked paprika and 6 roughly chopped tomatoes. Cook for 2 minutes. Add 300 ml (½ pint) chicken stock and a 400 g (13 oz) can cannellini beans, rinsed and drained. Bring to the boil and reduce the heat. Simmer for 3 minutes, add the chipolatas with the parsley and stir. Blend 1 tablespoon cornflour with 3 tablespoons water and add to the pan, stirring until thickened. Serve with crusty bread.

3 **Sausages and Peppers with Smoky Tomato Gravy** Place 8 large sausages in a roasting tin with 2 tablespoons olive oil and toss well to coat. Place in a preheated oven, 200°C (400°F), Gas Mark 6, for 5 minutes. Meanwhile, cut 250 g (8 oz) butternut squash into small pieces and cut 1 red, 1 yellow and 1 green pepper into chunks. Add to the roasting tin with the sausages and toss in the oil using 2 wooden spoons. Season with pepper. Return to the oven for 20 minutes until the vegetables are tender and the sausages cooked through. Meanwhile, to make the tomato gravy, place 200 g (7 oz) canned chopped tomatoes in a saucepan with 300 ml (½ pint) chicken stock and bring to the boil. Season well with pepper and add 1 teaspoon Dijon mustard. Transfer to a food processor and whizz until smooth, then return to the pan and place on the heat. Blend 1 tablespoon cornflour and ½ teaspoon smoked paprika with 3 tablespoons water and add to the gravy, stirring continuously, until boiled and thickened. Add 1 tablespoon chopped parsley and stir. Serve the sausages and roasted vegetables on warmed serving plates with the tomato gravy spooned over.

ABC-DEF-GHI-JKL

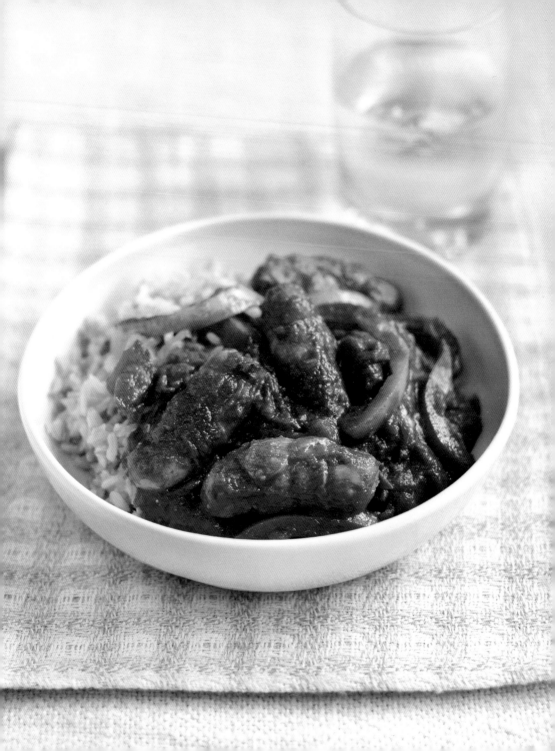

QuickCook
Tasty
Treats

Recipes listed by cooking time

30

20

10

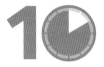 Strawberry and Raspberry Eton Mess

Serves 4

75 g (3 oz) strawberries, hulled
75 g (3 oz) raspberries
450 ml (¾ pint) double cream
4 meringue nests, broken into
   pieces

- Place the strawberries and raspberries in a bowl and lightly crush with a fork.

- Whip the cream in a separate bowl until just thick enough to form soft peaks. Lightly fold in the meringue pieces and the crushed fruit.

- Spoon into glasses or dishes to serve.

 Hot Berry Meringue Puddings

Using a fork, lightly crush 75 g (3 oz) hulled strawberries and 75 g (3 oz) raspberries with 1 tablespoon icing sugar and spoon into an ovenproof dish. In a clean bowl, whisk 2 egg whites until stiff, then whisk in 75 g (3 oz) caster sugar, 1 tablespoon at a time, whisking well after each addition until thick and glossy. Spoon the meringue mixture over the fruit and swirl with the back of the spoon. Bake in a preheated oven, 160°C (325°F), Gas Mark 3, for 10 minutes until golden. Dust with icing sugar and serve immediately.

 Floating Islands with Raspberries

Heat 500 ml (17 fl oz) milk in a saucepan until just below boiling point. Meanwhile mix together 1 tablespoon cornflour, 3 egg yolks and 75 g (3 oz) caster sugar. Slowly pour the hot milk over the egg yolk mixture, stirring continuously. Tip the mixture back into the pan and cook over a medium heat, stirring, until thick enough to coat the back of the spoon. In a separate bowl, whisk 3 egg whites until stiff, then gradually whisk in 75 g (3 oz) caster sugar. Drop spoonfuls of the meringue mixture into a saucepan of boiling water and cook for about 1 minute until they float. Remove with a slotted spoon and serve on top of the custard with a few raspberries.

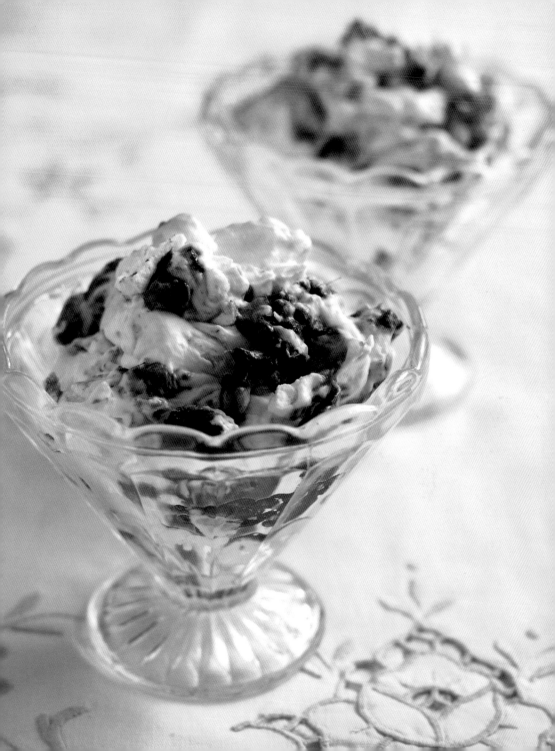

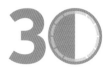

Peach and Brown Sugar Muffins

Makes 12

300 g (10 oz) self-raising flour
175 g (6 oz) light muscovado
  sugar, plus extra for sprinkling
½ teaspoon ground mixed spice
2 ripe peaches, stoned, each cut
  into 8 wedges and halved
  horizontally
150 g (5 oz) Greek yogurt
150 ml (¼ pint) milk
1 large egg
icing sugar, for dusting

- Line a 12-hole muffin tin with paper muffin cases.

- Place the flour, sugar and mixed spice in a bowl. Chop 20 of the peach pieces and add to the bowl.

- Mix together the yogurt, milk and egg in jug and add to the dry ingredients. Lightly stir until just combined – don't overmix.

- Spoon the mixture into the paper cases and push the remaining half-wedges of peach into the mixture. Sprinkle over a little sugar and bake in a preheated oven, 190°C (375°F), Gas Mark 5, for 15–20 minutes until well risen and golden. Remove to a wire rack and dust with icing sugar, before serving.

Peaches and Cream Muffins

Slice 4 ready-made muffins each into 3 slices horizontally. Whip 150 ml (¼ pint) double cream with ½ teaspoon ground mixed spice until just thick enough to form soft peaks, and thinly slice 1 peach. Sandwich the muffins back together with a spoonful of cream and a few slices of peach between the layers.

Peach and Brown Sugar Croissants

Unroll a 250 g (8 oz) can croissant dough and divide into 6 triangles along the perforations. Mix ½ teaspoon ground mixed spice with 50 g (2 oz) demerara sugar and sprinkle over the dough. Finely chop 1 ripe peach and sprinkle over the sugar. Roll up the croissants and bake in a preheated oven, 200°C (400°F), Gas Mark 6, for 10–12 minutes until well risen and golden.

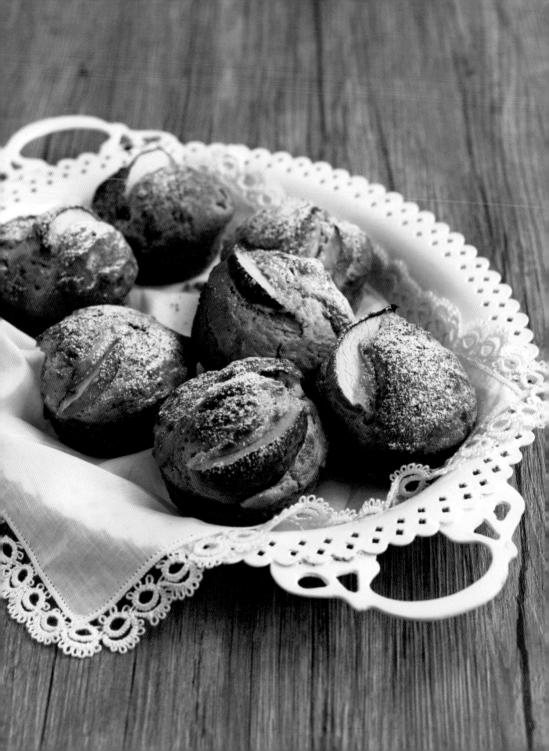

30 Blueberry Scones

Makes 6

250 g (8 oz) self-raising flour, plus extra for dusting
pinch of salt
50 g (2 oz) butter
25 g (1 oz) caster sugar
125 g (4 oz) blueberries
2 teaspoons lemon juice
150 ml (¼ pint) milk, plus extra for brushing
honey, to serve

- Line a baking sheet with baking paper.

- Place the flour and salt in a bowl and rub in the butter using your fingertips until the mixture resembles fine breadcrumbs. Stir in the sugar and blueberries.

- Mix the lemon juice with the milk and pour over the dry ingredients. Quickly mix using a round-bladed knife to form a soft dough, adding a little extra milk if the dough is too dry. Turn out on to a floured surface and very lightly knead a few times, then shape into a round, patting it out with your hands to about 1.5 cm (¾ inch) thick.

- Cut into 6 wedges, place on the baking sheet and brush the tops with milk. Bake in a preheated oven, 220°C (425°F), Gas Mark 7, for 10–12 minutes until well risen and golden.

- Cool slightly and serve warm, split and spread with honey.

---

1 Blueberry Drop Scones

Beat together 125 g (4 oz) self-raising flour, 2 teaspoons caster sugar, 1 egg, 1 tablespoon melted butter and 150 ml (¼ pint) milk to make a thick batter. Stir in 125 g (4 oz) blueberries. Drop spoonfuls on to a preheated, lightly greased frying pan and cook about 4 at a time for 2 minutes until bubbles appear. Turn the scones and cook for a further minute. Repeat with the remaining mixture. Serve warm with maple syrup.

2 Blueberry Scone Twists

Place a 320 g (11 oz) packet scone mix in a bowl. Stir in 125 g (4 oz) blueberries and make up with milk according to the packet instructions. Knead very lightly, then pat out the dough with your hands on a floured surface to a square about 1 cm (½ inch) thick. Sprinkle the surface with 25 g (1 oz) demerara sugar and cut into 8 strips. Twist the strips and place on a baking sheet lined with baking paper. Lightly brush with milk and bake in a preheated oven, 220°C (425°F), Gas Mark 7, for 10–12 minutes until well risen and golden. Serve warm or cold.

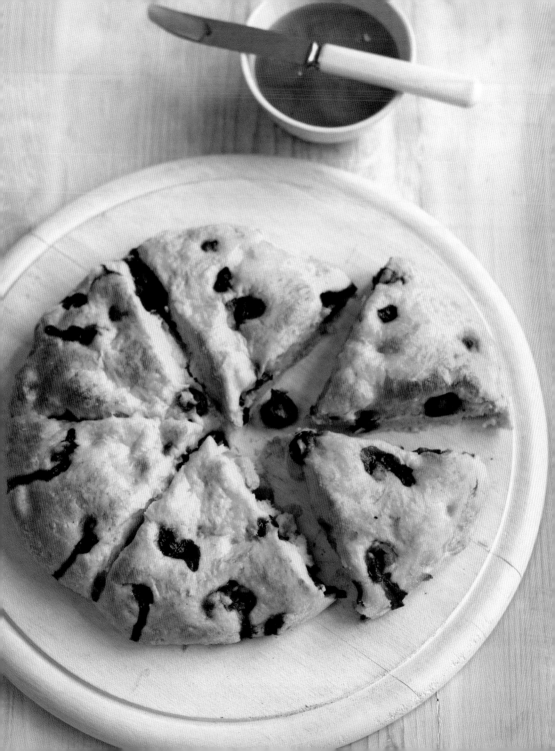

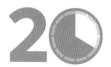

Wholemeal Pancakes with Peaches and Ice Cream

Serves 4

125 g (4 oz) wholemeal flour (or
  half wholemeal and half plain
  white flour)
pinch of salt
1 egg
15 g (½ oz) butter, melted
150 ml (¼ pint) milk
sunflower oil, for frying
3 ripe peaches, stoned and sliced,
  or sliced canned peaches
4 scoops of vanilla ice cream
4 tablespoons maple syrup

- Place the flour and salt in a mixing bowl. Make a well in the centre and break the egg into it. Add the melted butter and a quarter of the milk. Mix with a wooden spoon or hand whisk, adding more milk as the mixture thickens until all the milk is used. Beat well to make a smooth batter.

- Heat a small nonstick frying pan until hot and lightly grease with a little sunflower oil. Pour in about 2 tablespoons of batter, swirling the pan, so the batter evenly coats the bottom of the pan. Cook for 1 minute until golden underneath, then turn over and cook the other side until golden. Slide out on to a plate and keep warm. Repeat with the remaining batter to make 8 pancakes.

- Fold the pancakes into quarters and serve with the peach slices, a scoop of ice cream and a drizzle of maple syrup.

10 Waffles with Toffee Peaches and Cream

Heat 50 g (2 oz) butter, 150 g (5 oz) light muscovado sugar and 175 g (6 oz) can evaporated milk in a small saucepan until the butter has melted and the sugar dissolved. Bring to the boil and simmer gently for 3 minutes until the mixture has thickened slightly. Stir in 2 sliced peaches and serve with warmed ready-made waffles and a spoonful of extra-thick cream.

30 Peach Popovers

Beat together 125 g (4 oz) plain flour, a pinch of salt, 1 egg, 250 ml (8 fl oz) milk and 2 tablespoons caster sugar to make a smooth batter. Place 1 teaspoon sunflower oil in each cup of a 12-hole nonstick muffin tin and heat in a preheated oven, 220°C (425°F), Gas Mark 7, for 5 minutes. Cut 1 peach into 12 wedges and place a wedge of peach in each muffin hole. Quickly pour in the batter, dividing it equally between the holes, and cook in the oven for 15 minutes until well risen, crisp and golden. Turn out of the tins and serve warm, drizzled with maple syrup, with a scoop of ice cream.

KID-TAST-XOB

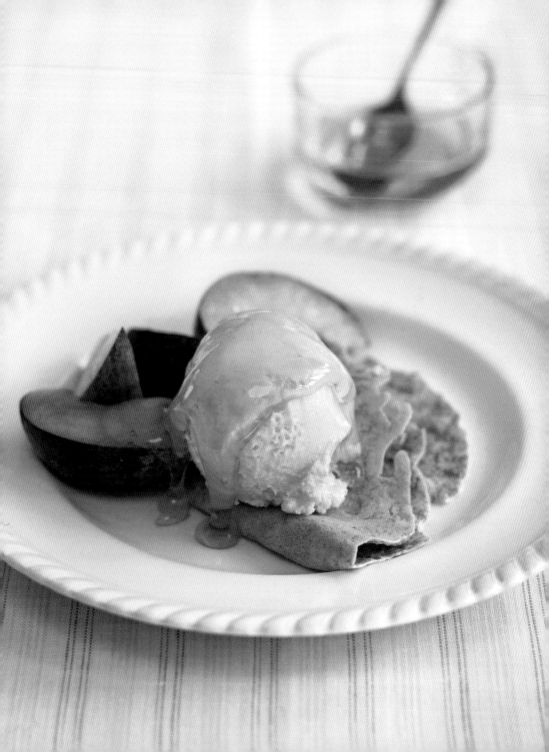

10 Chocolate Pots with Hidden Prunes

Serves 4

100 (3½ oz) plain dark chocolate, broken into pieces, plus extra shavings to decorate

400 g (13 oz) can prunes in apple juice, drained

300 g (10 oz) Greek yogurt

raspberries, to decorate

- Place the chocolate in a small microwave-proof bowl and melt in a microwave on medium for 1 minute. Stir and return to the microwave, checking every 20 seconds, until melted and smooth.

- Remove the stones from the prunes and whizz the flesh in a food processor or with a hand-held blender until smooth. Stir together the prune purée, yogurt and chocolate until evenly mixed.

- Spoon into cups or glasses and decorate with chocolate shavings and some raspberries.

 Chocolate and Prune Fools

Cook 150 g (5 oz) ready-to-eat pitted dried prunes in 100 ml (3½ fl oz) apple juice in a small saucepan for 5 minutes until soft. Purée with a hand-held blender until smooth. Stir through 250 ml (8 fl oz) natural yogurt with 50 g (2 oz) melted plain dark chocolate. Layer in glasses, alternating with 425 g (14 oz) ready-made custard.

 Hot Chocolate Prune Puddings

Using an electric whisk, beat together 125 g (4 oz) softened butter and 75 g (3 oz) light muscovado sugar until soft. Gradually whisk in 2 eggs, 200 g (7 oz) melted plain dark chocolate and 100 ml (3½ fl oz) double cream. Lightly fold in 25 g (1 oz) plain flour, ¼ teaspoon baking powder and 125 g (4 oz) chopped pitted ready-to-eat dried prunes. Spoon the mixture into 4 individual buttered ramekin dishes. Bake at 200°C (400°F), Gas Mark 6. leave to stand for 2 minutes before turning out. Serve warm with cream.

KID-TAST-MIX

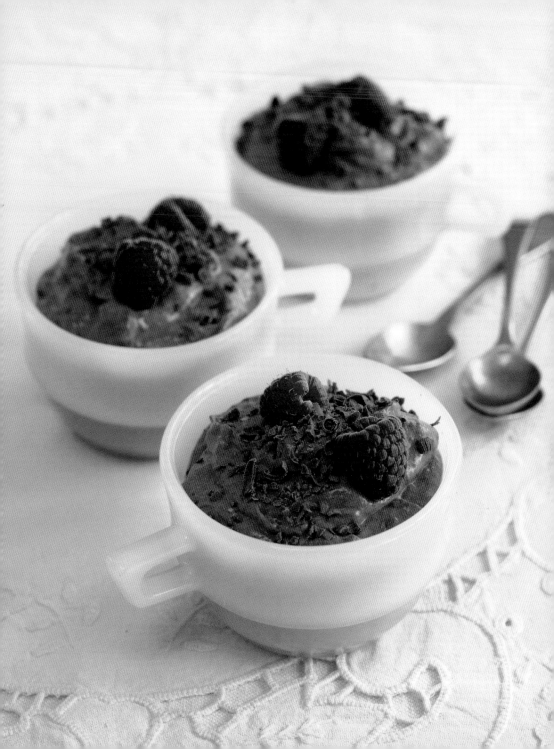

10 Fruit and Yogurt Baskets

Serves 4

2 tablespoons runny honey
300 g (10 oz) Greek yogurt
4 brandy snap baskets
300 g (10 oz) mixed fruits, such
  as strawberries, kiwifruit,
  apricots and grapes, halved or
  chopped depending on the fruit

- Lightly swirl the honey through the yogurt and spoon into the brandy snap baskets.

- Arrange the fruits on top and serve.

---

2 Fruity Yogurt Trifles

Using a fork, lightly crush 150 g (5 oz) hulled strawberries and 150 g (5 oz) blueberries. Sprinkle with 2 teaspoons icing sugar and leave to stand for 5 minutes until juicy. Break 8 sponge fingers into pieces and place in the bottom of 4 glasses or dishes. Spoon the crushed fruit on top with the juice and top with 1 sliced banana. Swirl 2 tablespoons runny honey into 300 g (10 oz) Greek yogurt and spoon over the fruit. Decorate with strawberry slices and blueberries.

3 Fruit and Yogurt Fool with Homemade Biscuits

Beat 125 g (4 oz) softened butter and 50 g (2 oz) caster sugar in a food processor. Add 175 g (6 oz) self-raising flour and whizz until the mixture just comes together and forms a dough. Divide the dough into 12 balls, place on a baking sheet lined with baking paper and flatten with the back of a wet fork. Bake in a preheated oven, 190°C (375°F), Gas Mark 5, for 10–12 minutes. Meanwhile, blend 150 g (5 oz) hulled strawberries and 150 g (5 oz) blueberries in a food processor until almost smooth. Fold into 150 g (5 oz) Greek yogurt, 150 g (5 oz) ready-made custard and 2 tablespoons runny honey to give a rippled effect. Spoon into glasses or bowls and serve with the biscuits.

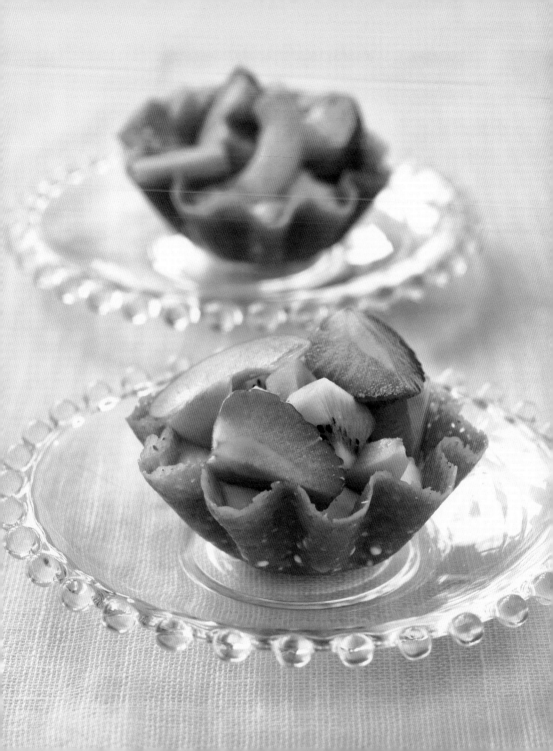

30 Apricot Oat Bars

Makes 15

250 g (8 oz) butter, plus extra for greasing

175 g (6 oz) golden syrup

175 g (6 oz) light muscovado sugar

400 g (13 oz) porridge oats

50 g (2 oz) crunchy mixed-grain cereal

175 g (6 oz) ready-to-eat dried apricots, chopped

- Grease a shallow 18 x 28 cm (7 x 11 inch) nonstick baking tin.

- Place the butter, golden syrup and sugar in a large saucepan and heat gently, stirring, until the butter has melted.

- Add the oats, cereal and apricots and stir well to mix. Tip the mixture into the baking tin and spread evenly.

- Bake in a preheated oven, 180°C (350°F), Gas Mark 4, for 15–20 minutes until golden. Cut into 15 bars, cool slightly, then remove from the tin. The bars can be stored in an airtight container for up to 5 days.

 1 Apricot and Fig Nibbles

Put 150 g (5 oz) ready-to-eat dried apricots in a food processor with 125 g (4 oz) ready-to-eat dried figs and pulse until chopped. Tip the chopped fruit into a bowl and stir in 125 g (4 oz) bran flakes, 75 g (3 oz) desiccated coconut, 250 ml (8 fl oz) condensed milk and 75 g (3 oz) melted butter. Spoon into 16 paper cake cases and eat or chill until set.

 2 Apricot Muesli Cookies

Melt 100 g (3½ oz) butter in a saucepan with 1 tablespoon golden syrup. Mix 1 teaspoon bicarbonate of soda with 2 tablespoons boiling water and add to the pan. Pour this mixture on to 175 g (6 oz) muesli, 100 g (3½ oz) plain flour, 100 g (3½ oz) caster sugar and 125 g (4 oz) chopped apricots. Stir well, then place 20 dessertspoonfuls of the mixture, allowing room for them to spread, on baking sheets lined with baking paper. Bake in a preheated oven, 180°C (350°F), Gas Mark 4, for 8–10 minutes.

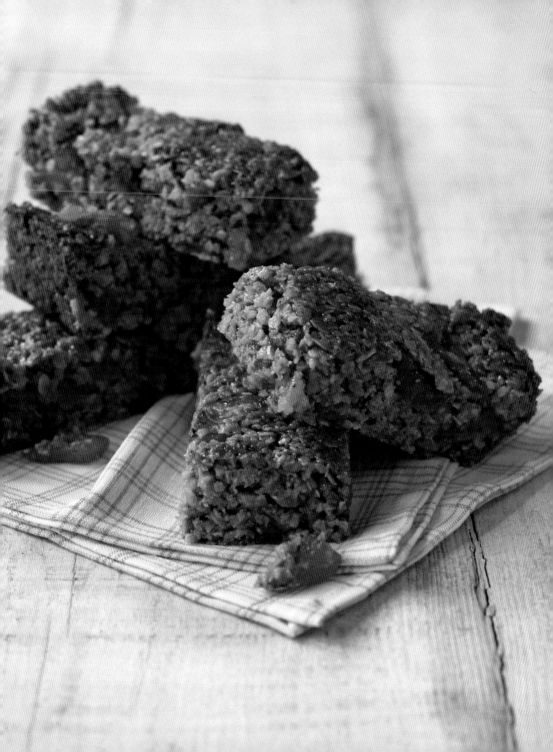

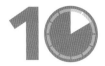

Strawberry Ice Cream Sundae

Serves 4

400 g (13 oz) strawberries, hulled
and quartered
50 g (2 oz) icing sugar
8 scoops of vanilla ice cream
50 g (2 oz) mini marshmallows
hundreds and thousands, to
decorate

- Blend half the strawberries with the icing sugar, using a hand-held blender or food processor, until smooth.

- Put 1 scoop of ice cream in the bottom of each of 4 tall glasses, top with half the remaining quartered strawberries, spoon over half the strawberry purée and sprinkle with half the marshmallows.

- Repeat the layers and finish with a sprinkle of hundreds and thousands. Serve immediately.

 Strawberry and Mallow Cookie Melts Thinly slice 4 hulled strawberries and arrange on the top of 4 chocolate chip cookies. Arrange mini marshmallows in a single layer on the top and cover each with another cookie. Wrap each cookie sandwich in foil, place on a baking sheet and bake in a preheated oven, 180°C (350°F), Gas Mark 4, for 5–8 minutes until the cookies are warm and the marshmallows have started to melt. Serve warm with a scoop of ice cream.

Mini Baked Alaskas Place 4 digestive biscuits on a baking sheet lined with baking paper. Top each biscuit with a scoop of strawberry ice cream and place in the freezer. Whisk 2 egg whites in a large clean bowl until stiff enough to form soft peaks. Gradually whisk in 125 g (4 oz) caster sugar, 1 tablespoon at a time, whisking well after each addition until thick and glossy. Quickly spread and swirl the meringue over the ice cream and biscuits, ensuring the ice cream is completely covered. Bake in a preheated oven, 220°C (425°F), Gas Mark 7, for 3–4 minutes until the meringue is golden. Dust with icing sugar and serve immediately before the ice cream starts to melt.

KID-TAST-XAY

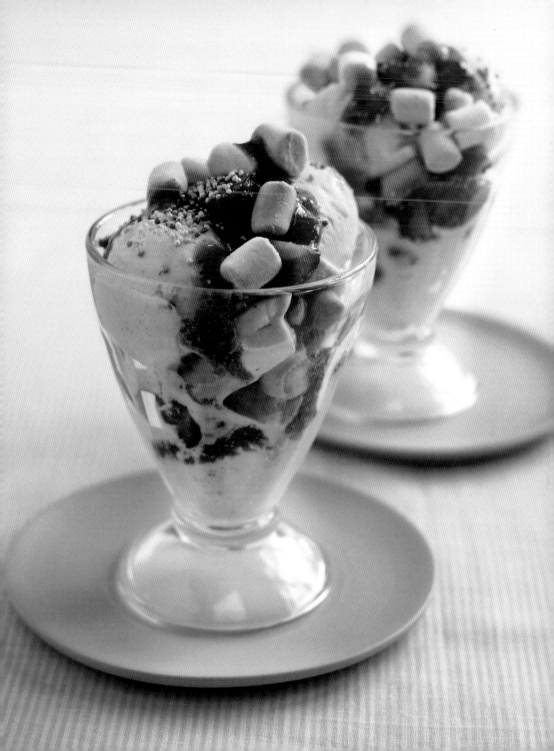

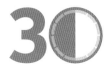 # Mango Krispie Cakes

Makes 16

50 g (2 oz) butter

3 tablespoons golden syrup

1 tablespoon light muscovado
  sugar

75 g (3 oz) Rice Krispies or similar
  cereal

75 g (3 oz) dried mango

50 g (2 oz) raisins

25 g (1 oz) pumpkin seeds

25 g (1 oz) sunflower seeds

- Melt the butter in a large saucepan over a low heat. Stir in the golden syrup and sugar and stir to dissolve the sugar.

- Remove from the heat, add the Rice Krispies, mango, raisins, pumpkin seeds and sunflower seeds and stir well to mix.

- Spoon the mixture into 16 paper cake cases and chill in the refrigerator for 15 minutes to set.

 Fruit, Seed and Krispie Mix

Mix together 75 g (3 oz) Rice Krispies or similar cereal, 75 g (3 oz) chopped dried mango, 50 g (2 oz) raisins, 25 g (1 oz) pumpkin seeds and 25 g (1 oz) sunflower seeds. Sprinkle over ice cream or yogurt, or simply eat as it is.

 Toffee Krispie Cakes

Unwrap a 200 g (7 oz) bag toffees and place in a saucepan with 4 tablespoons double cream. Slowly melt over a low heat, stirring occasionally, until smooth. Stir in 175 g (6 oz) Rice Krispies or similar cereal and 50 g (2 oz) chopped dried mango until evenly coated. Spoon into 20 paper cake cases.

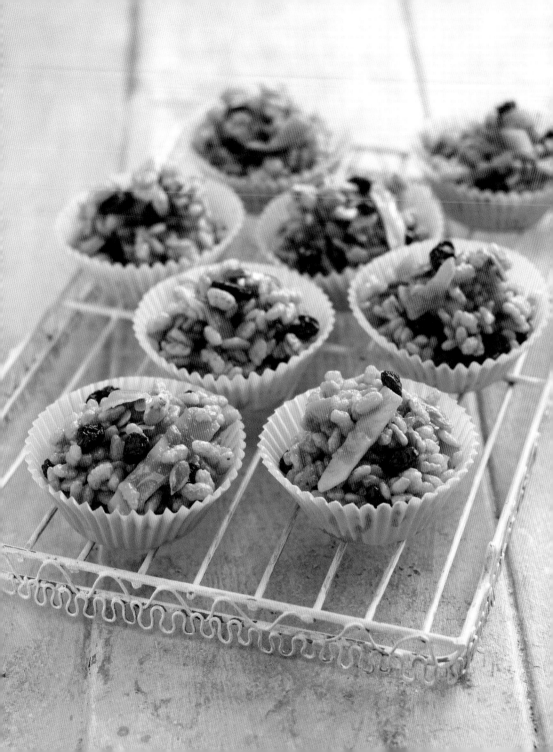

1️⃣0️⃣ Caramel Bananas

Serves 4

25 g (1 oz) butter
4 bananas, peeled and halved
  lengthways
6 tablespoons toffee sauce, such
  as dulce de leche
6 tablespoons double cream
ice cream, to serve

- Melt the butter in a large frying pan. Add the bananas and cook for 2 minutes, turning once, until just starting to soften and brown. Remove from the pan and place in serving dishes.

- Heat the toffee sauce and cream in the pan and simmer for 1 minute until bubbling. Leave to cool slightly.

- Drizzle the sauce over the bananas and serve with scoops of ice cream.

2️⃣0️⃣ Banana Fritters with Toffee Sauce

For the toffee sauce, heat 125 g (4 oz) butter and 125 g (4 oz) light muscovado sugar in a saucepan until the butter has melted and the sugar dissolved. Add 125 ml (4 fl oz) single cream and simmer for a few minutes until smooth and golden. Remove from the heat. For the fritters, mix together 125 g (4 oz) self-raising flour, 1 teaspoon bicarbonate of soda, 2 eggs and a splash of sparkling mineral water to make a smooth batter. Diagonally slice 2 large bananas and dip into the batter. Shake off the excess and fry, in batches, in hot oil (a pan half-filled with sunflower oil) for 2–3 minutes until crisp and golden. Remove from the pan with a slotted spoon and drain on kitchen paper. Serve warm with the toffee sauce.

3️⃣0️⃣ Banoffee Pie

Crush 250 g (8 oz) chocolate digestives in a food processor, then mix with 75 g (3 oz) melted butter. Press the biscuit mixture over the base and up the sides of a greased 20 cm (8 inch) round flan tin. Arrange 2 sliced bananas over the biscuit base and cover with 400 g (13 oz) toffee sauce, such as dulce de leche. Whip 300 ml (½ pint) whipping cream until just thick enough to form soft peaks, then swirl over the top of the caramel using the back of a spoon. Sprinkle grated chocolate over the top. Chill for 10 minutes to set the biscuits before serving.

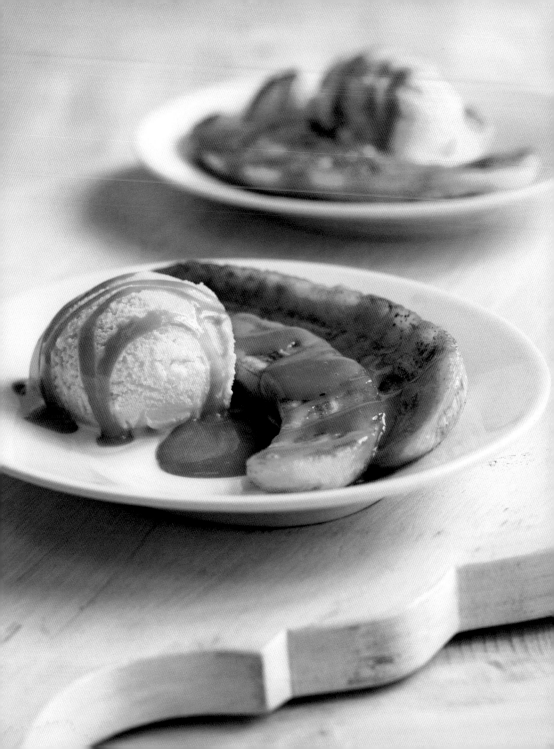

10 Rice Pudding and Jam Brûlée

Serves 4

4 tablespoons strawberry or raspberry jam

2 tablespoons orange juice

625 g (1¼ lb) canned creamed rice pudding

6 tablespoons demerara sugar

- Mix together the jam and orange juice and spoon into the base of 4 heatproof dishes.

- Spoon the rice pudding over the top and sprinkle evenly with the sugar.

- Place the puddings under a preheated hot grill, as near to the heat as possible, and grill for 2–3 minutes until the sugar is melted and bubbling. Leave for a few minutes for the topping to cool and set before eating.

---

20 Caramelized Blackberry Yogurt

Pots Place 150 g (5 oz) blackberries in a bowl and mash with a fork until broken into chunky pieces. Add the finely grated rind and juice of 1 orange and 1 tablespoon caster sugar and stir to mix. Divide between 4 x 175 ml (6 fl oz) individual heatproof dishes. Whip 150 ml (¼ pint) double cream until just thick enough to form soft peaks, then stir in 200 ml (7 fl oz) Greek yogurt. Spoon over the blackberries and level the tops just below the rim of each dish. Sprinkle 2 tablespoons caster sugar evenly over the top of each dish. Place under a preheated hot grill, as near to the heat as possible, and grill for 2–3 minutes until the sugar melts and turns golden, making sure it doesn't burn. Leave to cool until the caramel has set and cooled before serving.

---

30 Honey Baked Fruit with Brûlée

Topping Cut 4 ripe peaches in half and place in an ovenproof dish with 16 blackberries or 8 hulled strawberries, halved if large. Dot with a little butter and drizzle over 2 tablespoons clear honey. Bake in a preheated oven, 190°C (375°F), Gas Mark 5, for 20 minutes until softened. Spoon 250 g (8 oz) mascarpone cheese over the top, sprinkle with 6 tablespoons demerara sugar and cook under a preheated hot grill until the sugar starts to melt and bubble. Cool for 5 minutes before serving.

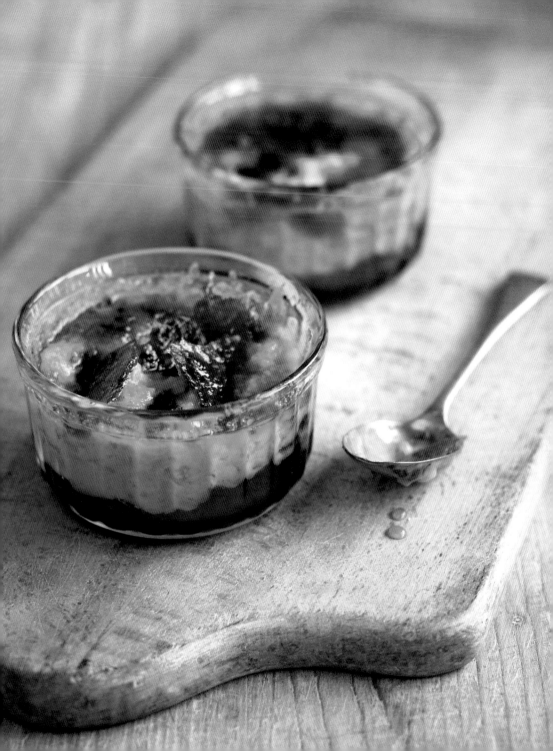

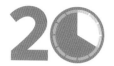

Rhubarb and Strawberry Oat Crumble

Serves 4

500 g (1 lb) rhubarb, trimmed and cut into 1 cm (½ inch) chunks
3 tablespoons water
75 g (3 oz) butter
175 g (6 oz) porridge oats
75 g (3 oz) demerara sugar
4 tablespoons strawberry jam
125 g (4 oz) strawberries, hulled and sliced
custard, to serve

- Place the rhubarb in a saucepan with the measurement water and cook for 5 minutes until soft.

- Meanwhile, in a separate saucepan, melt the butter, then stir in the oats and sugar.

- Stir the jam into the rhubarb, add the sliced strawberries, then tip into an ovenproof dish. Sprinkle over the oat mixture and bake in a preheated oven, 200 °C (400 °F), Gas Mark 6, for 15 minutes until golden.

- Serve warm with custard.

Rhubarb and Summer Fruit Shortcake Crumbles Cut 300 g (10 oz) rhubarb into 1 cm (½ inch) chunks and cook in a saucepan with 25 g (1 oz) butter for 5 minutes, stirring occasionally, until softened. Stir in 450 g (14½ oz) ready-made summer fruit compote and heat through. Spoon into bowls and sprinkle with 175 g (6 oz) crumbled shortcake biscuits. Serve warm with custard.

Nutty Rhubarb and Strawberry Crumble Cut 500 g (1 lb) rhubarb into 1 cm (½ inch) chunks and place in a large baking dish with 250 g (8 oz) strawberries, hulled and halved. Sprinkle over 75 g (3 oz) caster sugar and bake in a preheated oven, 200 °C (400 °F), Gas Mark 6, for 10 minutes. Meanwhile, place 175 g (6 oz) plain flour in a food processor with 125 g (4 oz) butter and 75 g (3 oz) demerara sugar. Pulse until the mixture forms fine breadcrumbs. Tip into a bowl and stir in 75 g (3 oz) chopped hazelnuts. Rub the crumbs together until they start to form clumps, sprinkle over the fruit and return to the oven for 15 minutes until the crumble is golden. Serve warm with custard.

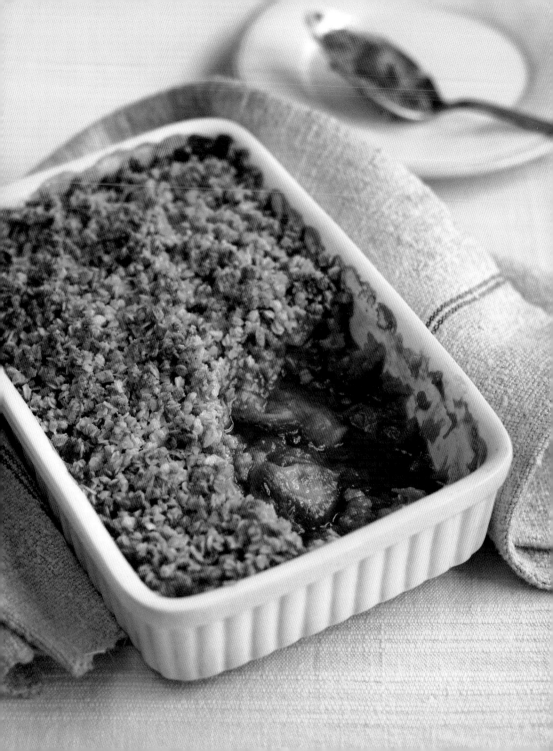

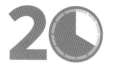

20 White Chocolate and Apricot Squares

Makes 9

250 g (8 oz) white chocolate, broken into pieces

65 g (2½ oz) Rice Krispies

50 g (2 oz) ready-to-eat dried apricots, chopped

- Line a shallow 20 cm (8 inch) square baking tin with clingfilm.

- Heat 200g (7 oz) of the white chocolate in a heatproof bowl over a saucepan of simmering water, making sure the base of the bowl doesn't touch the water. Leave for a few minutes, stirring occasionally, until the chocolate is melted and smooth.

- Remove the bowl from the pan and stir the Rice Krispies and apricots into the melted chocolate. Spoon the mixture into the prepared tin and press down firmly. Chop the remaining 50 g (2 oz) chocolate and scatter over the top. Place in the freezer for 15 minutes to chill and set.

- Cut into 9 squares to serve.

 White Chocolate and Apricot Popcorn Stir 100 g (3½ oz) sweet popcorn into 75 g (3 oz) melted white chocolate with 50 g (2 oz) chopped ready-to-eat dried apricots. Spoon into small paper cones or cake cases and chill in the freezer for 5 minutes to set.

 White Chocolate and Fruit Fridge Cake Melt 200 g (7 oz) white chocolate, broken into pieces, 75 g (3 oz) butter and 2 tablespoons golden syrup in a heatproof bowl over a saucepan of simmering water. Stir until melted, then remove from the heat and stir in 75 g (3 oz) broken digestive biscuits, 25 g (1 oz) cornflakes, 50 g (2 oz) raisins, 75 g (3 oz) chopped ready-to-eat dried apricots and 50 g (2 oz) dried cranberries. Mix well, then spoon into a shallow 20 cm (8 inch) square cake tin lined with clingfilm. Place in the freezer for 20 minutes to chill and set. Cut into squares.

KID-TAST-GUD

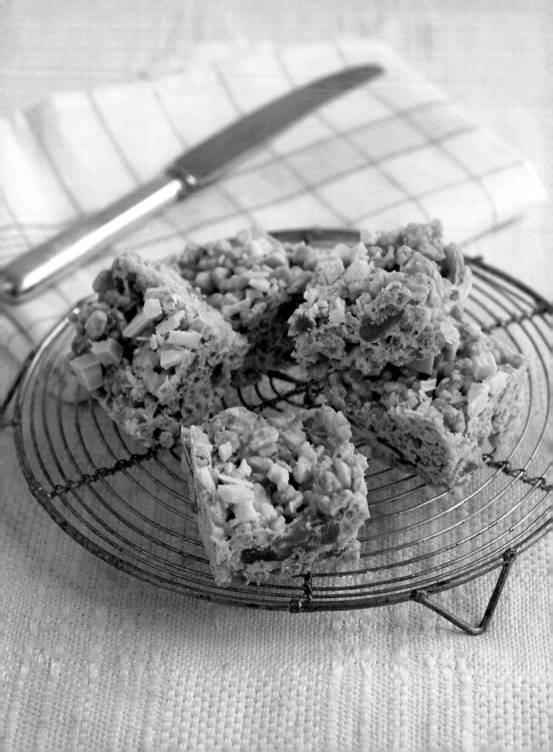

3⊘ Apple and Almond Tart

Serves 6

325 g (11 oz) ready-rolled
   puff pastry
250 g (8 oz) marzipan, coarsely
   grated
2 red-skinned dessert apples,
   cored and thinly sliced
4 tablespoons apricot jam,
   warmed
50 g (2 oz) flaked almonds
cream or ice cream, to serve

- Unroll the puff pastry and place on a baking sheet. Sprinkle the grated marzipan evenly over, then arrange the apple slices in rows over the top.

- Brush the apricot jam over the apple slices and sprinkle with the flaked almonds. Bake in a preheated oven, 200°C (400°F), Gas Mark 6, for 20 minutes until the pastry is golden and cooked.

- Cut into squares and serve warm with cream or ice cream.

1⊘ Speedy Apple Pies Heat 375 g (12 oz) canned apple slices in 25 g (1 oz) butter in a frying pan, add ½ teaspoon ground cinnamon and 25 g (1 oz) sultanas and heat through, adding a little water if necessary. Spoon into dishes and place 1 ready-made palmier biscuit on top of each. Serve with cream.

2⊘ Hot Apple Slices with Cinnamon Pastries Unroll 325 g (11 oz) ready-rolled puff pastry. Mix 4 tablespoons caster sugar and 1 teaspoon ground cinnamon and sprinkle evenly over the pastry. Starting along one of the long sides, loosely roll the pastry into a long roll. Cut into 1 cm (½ inch) slices and lay flat on 2 baking sheets lined with baking paper. Sprinkle with a little extra sugar and bake in a preheated oven, 200°C (400°F), Gas Mark 6, for 10 minutes until golden and crisp. Meanwhile, fry 3 cored and sliced dessert apples in 25 g (1 oz) butter for 5 minutes until softened and starting to brown. Add 25 g (1 oz) sultanas. Serve with the cinnamon pastries.

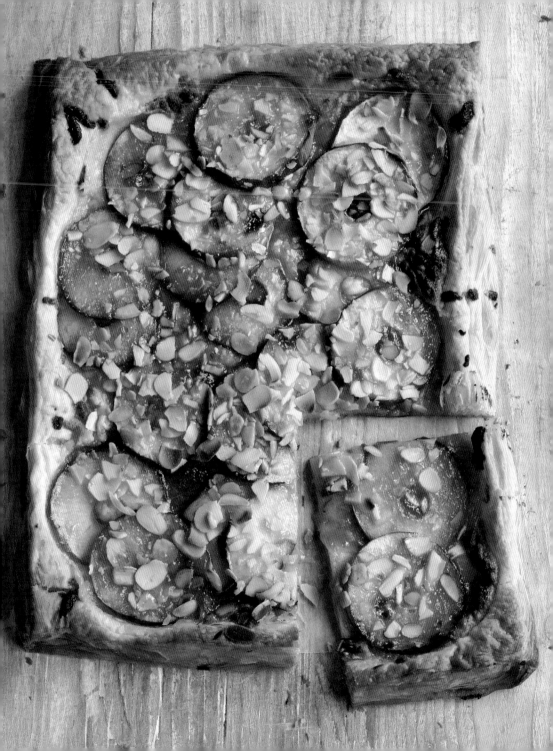

30 Strawberry and Lime Cheesecakes

Serves 4

100 g (3½ oz) oat biscuits, such as Hobnobs, crushed

50 g (2 oz) butter, melted

6 tablespoons condensed milk

250 g (8 oz) mascarpone cheese

finely grated rind and juice of 1 lime

125 g (4 oz) strawberries, hulled and sliced

1 tablespoon strawberry jam

- Mix together the crushed biscuits and butter and spoon into the base of 4 chunky glasses or ramekins. Press down firmly with the back of a small spoon.

- In a bowl, mix the condensed milk and mascarpone until soft and creamy. Stir in the lime rind and juice and spoon into the glasses. Place the glasses or ramekins in the refrigerator for 10 minutes to chill the desserts.

- Meanwhile, mix together the strawberries and jam (if the jam is very thick, soften it with a dash of boiling water from the kettle) and spoon over the top of the cheesecakes.

---

 1 Strawberry and Lime Cheesecake Stacks Mix 250 g (8 oz) mascarpone cheese with 175 g (6 oz) condensed milk and stir in the grated rind and juice of 1 lime. Slice 125 g (4 oz) hulled strawberries. Spoon half the mascarpone mixture on to 4 digestive biscuits and top with half the strawberries. Repeat the layers and finish with a dusting of icing sugar.

 2 Strawberry and Lime Tiramisu Place 8 sponge fingers in a single layer in the base of a dish. Arrange 50 g (2 oz) sliced hulled strawberries over the top and dust generously with icing sugar. Mix together 250 g (8 oz) mascarpone cheese, 175 g (6 oz) condensed milk and the grated rind and juice of 1 lime. Spread half the mixture over the strawberries, cover with 8 more sponge fingers, another 50 g (2 oz) sliced strawberries and a dusting of icing sugar. Spoon the remaining mascarpone mixture over the top, sprinkle with 25 g (1 oz) grated chocolate and decorate with extra strawberries.

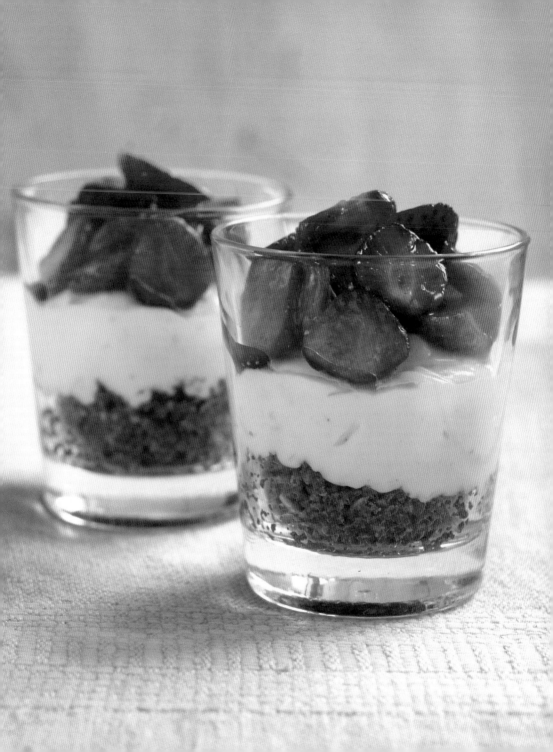

30 Orange Drizzle Tray Bake

Makes 12

125 g (4 oz) sunflower spread
125 g (4 oz) golden caster sugar,
   plus 4 tablespoons
125 g (4 oz) self-raising flour
2 eggs
finely grated rind and juice of
   1 orange
crystallized orange and lemon
   slices, to decorate

- Line a shallow 18 x 28 cm (7 x 11 inch) baking tin with baking paper.

- Place the sunflower spread, 125 g (4 oz) sugar, flour, eggs and orange rind in a mixing bowl and beat with an electric mixer until soft and creamy. Spoon the mixture into the tin and spread the surface level.

- Bake in a preheated oven, 180°C (350°F), Gas Mark 4, for 20 minutes until risen and just firm to the touch. Meanwhile, mix together the orange juice and remaining sugar in a bowl. Remove the cake from the oven and drizzle the mixture over the cake.

- Cut into 12 fingers or squares and top each with a crystallized orange and lemon slice.

---

1 Sticky Orange Syrup Cakes

Heat 4 tablespoons shredless marmalade in a small saucepan with 2 tablespoons water until melted and smooth, then bring to the boil. Remove from the heat. Spoon the syrup over 12 ready-made plain fairy cakes and leave to soak for a few minutes. Dust with icing sugar to serve.

2 Iced Orange Fairy Cakes

Using an electric mixer, beat 125 g (4 oz) sunflower spread, 125 g (4 oz) golden caster sugar, 125 g (4 oz) self-raising flour, 2 eggs and 2 tablespoons fine-cut orange marmalade until soft and creamy. Spoon into 12 paper cake cases and bake in a preheated oven, 180°C (350°F), Gas Mark 4, for 10 minutes until risen and just firm to the touch. Meanwhile, mix together 150 g (5 oz) icing sugar, the finely grated rind of ½ orange and enough orange juice to make a smooth, thick icing. Spoon the icing over the cakes.

KID-TAST-KOT

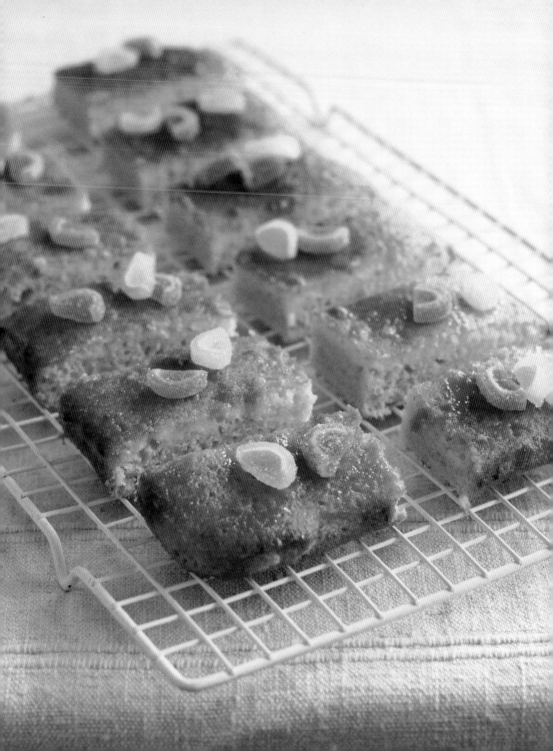

Cherry Clafouti

Serves 4

425 g (14 oz) can pitted black cherries, drained and dried on kitchen paper
125 g (4 oz) plain flour
50 g (2 oz) caster sugar
3 eggs
400 ml (14 fl oz) milk
icing sugar, for dusting

- Grease a baking dish then arrange the cherries in a single layer in the base.

- Beat together the flour, sugar, eggs and milk to make a smooth batter.

- Pour the batter over the cherries and bake in a preheated oven, 180°C (350°F), Gas Mark 4, for 25 minutes until golden and just set. Serve warm with a dusting of icing sugar.

 ### Fried Cherry Sandwiches

For each sandwich, butter 2 slices of bread, spread 1 slice with cherry jam and sandwich together. Beat 1 egg in a shallow bowl and dip both sides of the sandwich in it. Heat 25 g (1 oz) butter in a frying pan, add the sandwich and cook for 2 minutes until golden. Turn and cook the other side. Serve warm, dusted with icing sugar.

 ### Warm Cherry Pancakes

Heat 50 g (2 oz) caster sugar, 50 g (2 oz) butter and 4 tablespoons orange juice in a large frying pan until the butter has melted and the sugar dissolved. Drain a 425 g (14 oz) can pitted black cherries, reserving the juice. Mix the cherry juice with 1 tablespoon cornflour blended to a paste with 1 tablespoon cold water and pour into the pan. Bring to the boil, stirring, until thickened and smooth. Fold 4 ready-made pancakes into quarters and place in the pan with the sauce. Add the cherries and heat through for a few minutes, spooning some of the sauce over the pancakes. Serve with cream.

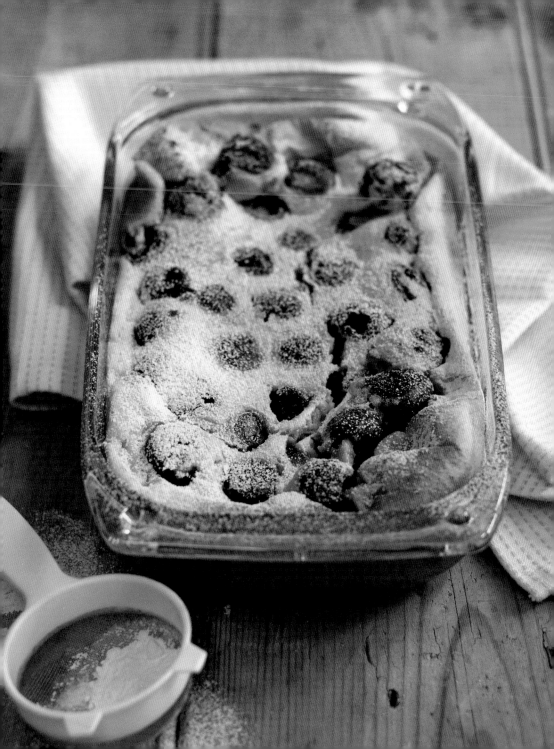

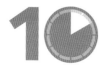

Chocolate-Dipped Fruits

Makes about 30

175 g (6 oz) plain dark or milk chocolate, broken into pieces
175 g (6 oz) white chocolate, broken into pieces
10 strawberries, with stalks on
1 banana, thickly sliced
10 pieces of canned pineapple

- Heat the plain or milk and white chocolate in separate heatproof bowls over separate saucepans of simmering water, making sure the bases of the bowl don't touch the water. Leave for a few minutes, stirring occasionally, until the chocolate is melted and smooth. Transfer the melted chocolates to 2 small cups or serving bowls.

- Stick the pieces of fruit on to cocktail sticks and dip into the warm chocolate. Either eat immediately or place on baking sheets lined with baking paper and chill for a few minutes until the chocolate sets.

 Iced Berries with Warm Chocolate Sauce Spread 300 g (10 oz) frozen mixed berries, such as raspberries, blackberries, redcurrants and blackcurrants, over a plate and allow to defrost slightly for 15 minutes. Meanwhile the fruit is defrosting, put 125 g (4 oz) plain dark, milk or white chocolate into a heatproof bowl with 150 ml (¼ pint) double cream. Place the bowl over a saucepan of simmering water and stir until the chocolate has melted and the sauce is smooth. Spoon the semi-frozen berries into glasses or dishes and serve with the warm chocolate sauce poured over.

 Warm Chocolate and Berry Tart Heat a 425 g (14 oz) can custard with 175 g (6 oz) plain dark chocolate, broken into pieces, in a saucepan over a low heat until the chocolate melts and the custard is smooth. Cool for 10 minutes, then pour into a ready-made sweet pastry case. Chop 250 g (8 oz) mixed summer fruits and spoon over the custard. Dust with icing sugar and serve.

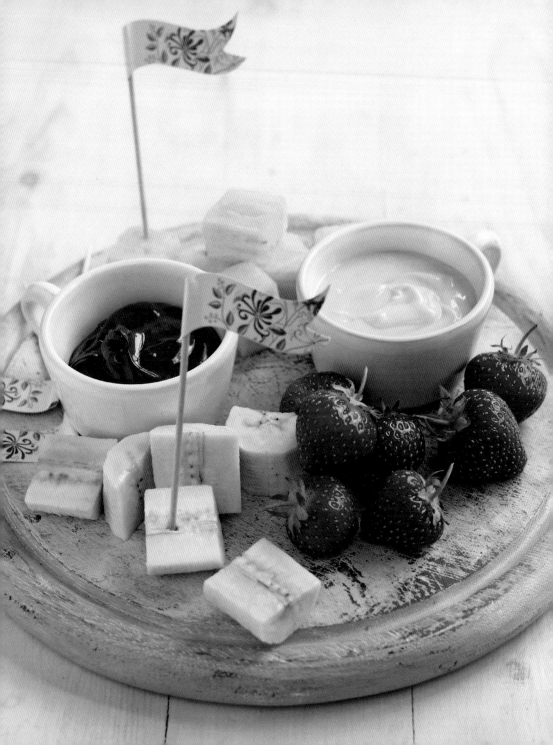

30 Iced Banana and Raspberry Cupcakes

Makes 12

125 g (4 oz) self-raising flour
1 teaspoon baking powder
25 g (1 oz) caster sugar
1 ripe banana, mashed
1 egg
1 tablespoon honey
50 g (2 oz) butter, melted
50 g (2 oz) raspberries, lightly
  crushed
50 g (2 oz) icing sugar
1–2 teaspoons water
pink food colouring
sugar flowers, to decorate

- Line a 12-hole bun tin with paper cake cases.

- Sift the flour and baking powder into a bowl and stir in the caster sugar. Mix together the mashed banana, egg, honey and melted butter in a separate bowl, then add to the dry ingredients. Stir in the raspberries until mixed.

- Spoon the mixture into the cake cases and bake in a preheated oven, 180°C (350°F), Gas Mark 4, for 15 minutes until golden and just firm to the touch. Leave to cool slightly.

- Mix the icing sugar with the measurement water to make a smooth icing. Add a drop of pink food colouring and stir to mix. Spoon on to the buns and decorate with sugar flowers.

10 Banana and Honey Frosted Cakes

Mix together 1 ripe mashed banana, 175 g (6 oz) full-fat soft cheese and 1 tablespoon honey. Spread over the top of ready-made plain fairy cakes and top each with a banana chip.

20 Banana and Honey Cakes

Make up a 300 g (10 oz) packet vanilla cupcake mix according to the packet instructions. Mash 1 ripe banana with a fork and stir into the cake mixture with 1 tablespoon honey. Spoon the mixture into paper cake cases and bake in a preheated oven, 180°C (350°F), Gas Mark 4, for 15 minutes. Brush with a little extra honey while warm and stick a banana chip on the top of each cake.

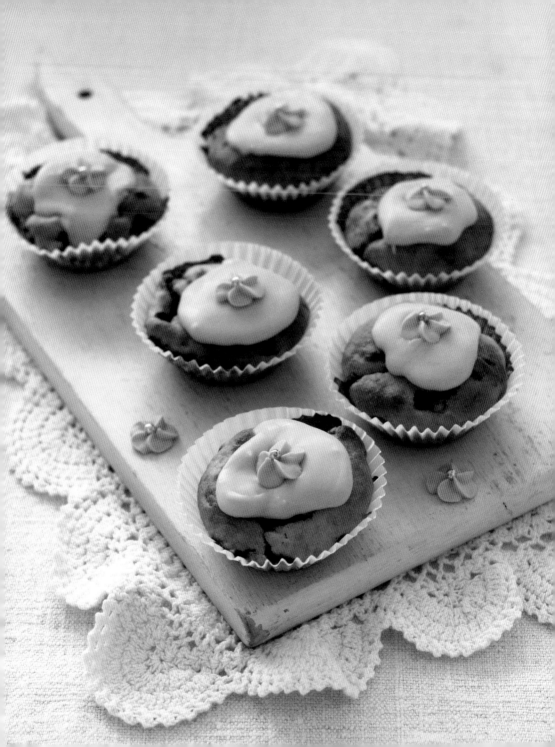

30 Saucy Lemon Puddings

Serves 4

butter, for greasing
1 egg, separated
40 g (1½ oz) caster sugar
1 tablespoon plain flour
finely grated rind and juice of
  1 lemon
125 ml (4 fl oz) milk
icing sugar, for dusting

- Lightly grease 4 ovenproof dishes or teacups, then stand them in a roasting tin.

- Place the egg yolk and caster sugar in a large bowl and whisk together, using an electric mixer, until creamy. Whisk in the flour, lemon rind and juice until smooth, then gradually whisk in the milk.

- In a separate clean bowl, whisk the egg white until soft peaks form. Lightly fold into the lemon mixture and spoon into the cups or dishes. Pour boiling water into the roasting tin to come halfway up the sides of the cups or dishes and bake in a preheated oven, 180°C (350°F), Gas Mark 4, for 15–20 minutes until risen and golden. The sauce will separate during cooking underneath the fluffy tops.

- Dust with icing sugar and serve immediately.

10 Madeira Cake with Lemon Custard

Pour 425 g (14 oz) ready-made custard into a microwave-proof jug and heat in the microwave on full power for 3 minutes. Stir in 4 tablespoons lemon curd and heat for a further minute on full power. Cut 4 thick slices of Madeira cake into chunks, spread out over a microwave-proof plate and heat on full power for 30 seconds until warm. Divide the cake between 4 bowls and pour over the warm custard.

20 Lemon Sponge Puddings

Place 4 individual ramekins in a roasting tray. Using an electric mixer, whisk together 125 g (4 oz) sunflower spread, 125 g (4 oz) caster sugar, 125 g (4 oz) self-raising flour and 2 eggs until soft and creamy. Spoon the mixture into the ramekins and pour boiling water to half-fill the roasting tray. Cook in a preheated oven, 180°C (350°F), Gas Mark 4, for 15 minutes. Heat 4 tablespoons lemon curd in the microwave for 30 seconds until warmed. Spoon over the sponge pudding and serve with custard or cream.

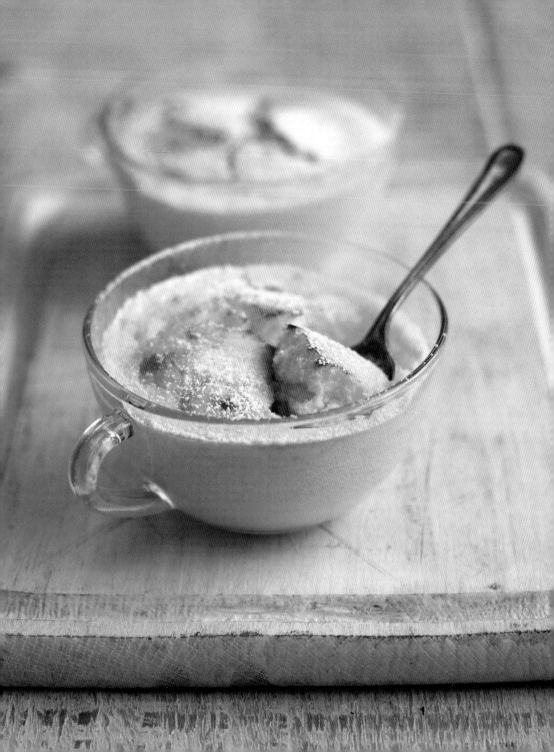

30 Chocolate Flapjacks

Makes 10

175 g (6 oz) butter, plus extra for greasing

1½ tablespoons golden syrup

175 g (6 oz) light muscovado sugar

300 g (10 oz) porridge oats

3 tablespoons good-quality cocoa powder

- Grease a shallow 20 cm (8 inch) square baking tin.

- Melt the butter, golden syrup and sugar in a saucepan over a low heat until just melted but not boiling. Remove from the heat and stir in the oats and cocoa powder.

- Press the mixture into the prepared tin and bake in a preheated oven, 150°C (300°F), Gas Mark 2, for 20 minutes.

- Leave to cool slightly, then cut into fingers.

 1 Crunchy Chocolate Oat Crumble

Melt 40 g (1½ oz) sunflower spread in a saucepan. Remove from the heat and stir in 25 g (1 oz) demerara sugar and 50 g (2 oz) porridge oats. Spread out over a foil-lined baking sheet and cook under a preheated hot grill for 2–3 minutes, stirring occasionally, until golden and crisp. Tip into a bowl and stir in 50 g (2 oz) chocolate chips. Sprinkle the mixture over sliced bananas, ready-made fruit compote or yogurt.

 2 Mini Chocolate Oat Bites

Place 125 g (4 oz) sunflower spread in a microwave-proof bowl with 50 g (2 oz) light muscovado sugar and 2 tablespoons clear honey. Heat in the microwave on full power for 30 seconds until just melted. Stir in 125 g (4 oz) porridge oats, 125 g (4 oz) self-raising flour, ½ teaspoon ground mixed spice and 50 g (2 oz) chocolate chips. Place about 30 heaped teaspoons of the mixture on 2 baking sheets lined with baking paper and bake in a preheated oven, 180°C (350°F), Gas Mark 4, for 10 minutes until golden. Eat warm or cold.

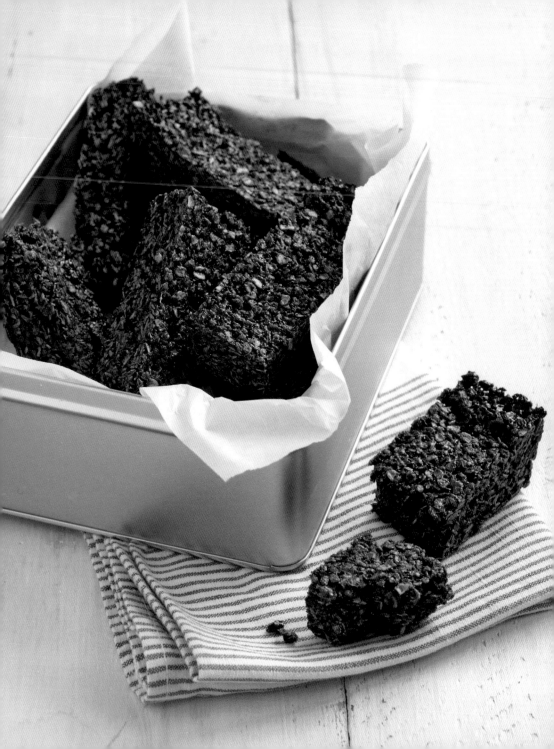

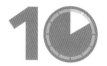 # Quick Summer Fruit Ice Cream

Serves 4

500 g (1 lb) frozen summer fruits
50 g (2 oz) icing sugar
1 tablespoon clear honey
400 g (13 oz) can custard
sugar strands, to decorate

- Reserve a few of the fruits for decoration. Place the remaining fruits in a food processor with the icing sugar and honey and blend until smooth.

- While the motor is running, slowly pour in the custard until the mixture is thick and forms a soft ice cream.

- Spoon into paper cups or bowls, then sprinkle with sugar strands before serving.

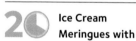 **Ice Cream Meringues with Summer Fruit Sauce** Place 500 g (1 lb) frozen summer fruits in a saucepan with 50g (2 oz) icing sugar. Heat, stirring, until the fruits have defrosted. Tip the fruits and their juice into a food processor and blend until smooth. Add a little water if the mixture is too thick and blend again until the sauce is smooth. Place scoops of ice cream on ready-made meringue nests and serve with the fruit sauce.

 Iced Summer Fruit Meringue Bombes Blend 500 g (1 lb) frozen summer fruits in a food processor with 50 g (2 oz) icing sugar and a 400 g (13 oz) can custard. Tip into a bowl and quickly stir in 3 crushed meringue nests. Spoon the mixture into 6 clingfilm-lined individual pudding basins or ramekins. Freeze for 20 minutes, then turn out, remove the clingfilm and serve with raspberries.

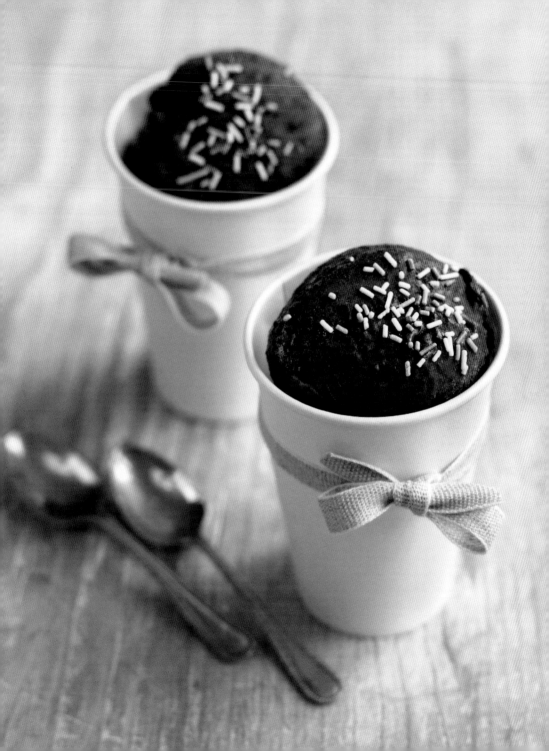

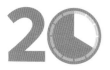

Spiced Raisin and Cranberry Cookies

Makes 8

125 g (4 oz) butter

125 g (4 oz) light muscovado sugar

1 tablespoon golden syrup

125 g (4 oz) self-raising flour

½ teaspoon ground mixed spice

125 g (4 oz) porridge oats

50 g (2 oz) raisins

50 g (2 oz) dried cranberries

- Line 2 baking sheets with baking paper.

- Heat the butter, sugar and golden syrup in a saucepan until just melted. Remove from the pan and stir in the flour, mixed spice, oats and fruit.

- Roll the mixture into 8 balls, place on the prepared baking sheets and flatten slightly. Bake in a preheated oven, 180°C (350°F), Gas Mark 4, for 10–12 minutes.

 Raisin Cookie and Cranberry Sundaes

Break 5 ready-made oat and raisin cookies into pieces and sprinkle over scoops of soft vanilla ice cream in glasses. Top with a sprinkling of dried cranberries.

 Spiced Cranberry and Raisin Cupcakes In a food processor, blend 125 g (4 oz) self-raising flour, ½ teaspoon ground mixed spice, 125 g (4 oz) sunflower spread, 125 g (4 oz) caster sugar and 2 eggs until smooth and creamy. Stir in 1 finely chopped dessert apple, 75 g (3 oz) raisins and 25 g (1 oz) dried cranberries. Spoon into 12 paper cake cases and bake in a preheated oven, 180°C (350°F), Gas Mark 4, for 15–20 minutes.

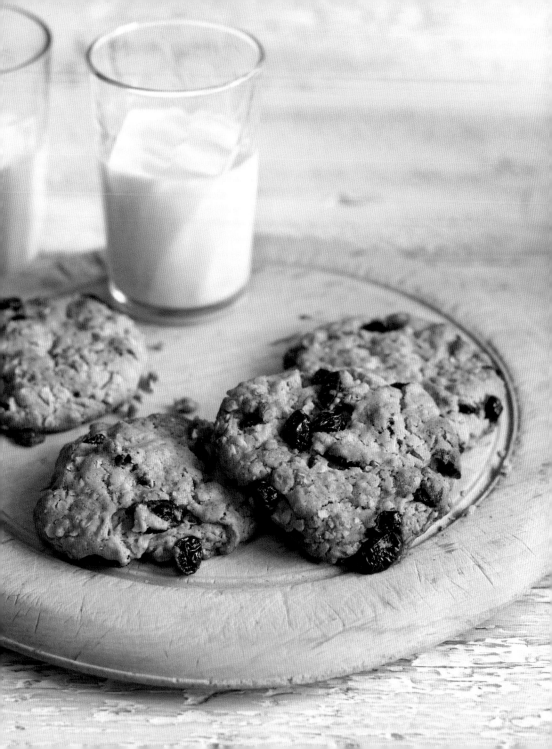

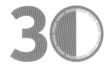

30 Wheat-Free Gooey Chocolate Brownies

Makes 16

200 g (7 oz) plain dark chocolate, broken into pieces

125 g (4 oz) unsalted butter, softened

275 g (9 oz) light muscovado sugar

4 eggs, beaten

1 teaspoon vanilla extract

50 g (2 oz) ground almonds

50 g (2 oz) cocoa powder

- Line a shallow 23 cm (9 inch) square cake tin with baking paper.

- Heat the chocolate and butter in a heatproof bowl over a pan of simmering water, making sure the base of the bowl doesn't touch the water, until melted and smooth. Remove from the heat and cool slightly.

- Add the sugar and beat together. Gradually beat in the eggs and vanilla extract to the melted chocolate mixture. Add the ground almonds, sift in the cocoa powder and stir well to mix.

- Spoon the mixture into the prepared tin and bake in a preheated oven, 180°C (350°F), Gas Mark 4, for 20 minutes until just firm to the touch but still a bit soft. Leave to cool slightly before cutting into 16 squares.

---

10 Wheat-Free Brownies with Warm Chocolate Fudge Sauce

In a small saucepan gently heat 50 g (2 oz) light muscovado sugar, 50 g (2 oz) butter, 75 ml (3 fl oz) double cream and 75 g (3 oz) plain dark chocolate, broken into pieces. Stir occasionally until the chocolate has melted, the sugar has dissolved and the sauce is smooth. Pour over ready-made wheat-free brownies and serve with a scoop of ice cream.

20 Wheat-Free Mars Bar Krispie Bites

Chop 2 Mars Bars and place in a heatproof bowl with 50 g (2 oz) butter over a saucepan of simmering water. Stir occasionally until the mixture is melted and smooth. Remove from the heat and stir in 50 g (2 oz) Rice Krispies, or similar cereal, until evenly coated. Place spoonfuls of the mixture on a baking sheet lined with baking paper and chill in the freezer for 10 minutes to set.

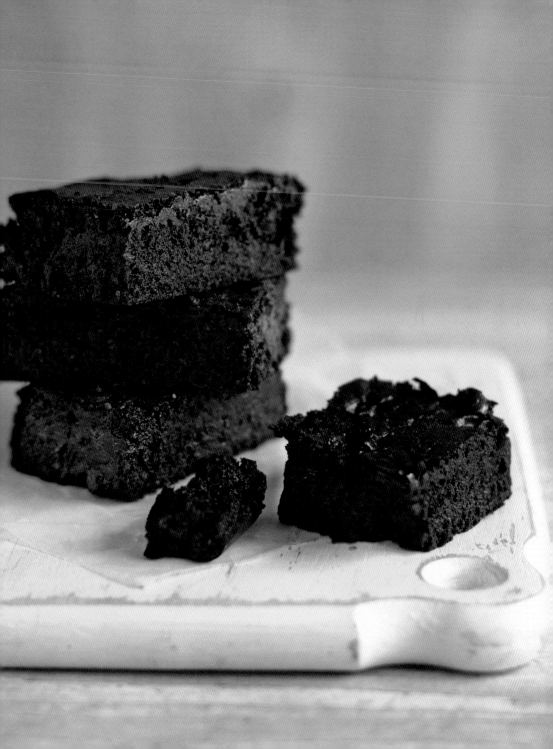

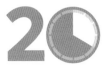

Chocolate Muffin and Custard Trifles

Serves 4

400 g (13 oz) can custard

125 g (4 oz) milk chocolate, broken into pieces

2 chocolate muffins, broken into chunks

400 g (13 oz) can black cherry pie filling

150 ml (¼ pint) whipping cream

1 small chocolate flake, broken into pieces

- Heat the custard iand chocolate in a small saucepan over a low heat, stirring, until the chocolate melts and the custard is smooth. Leave to cool slightly.

- Divide the muffins between 4 glasses or bowls, or 1 large bowl, and spoon the cherry pie filling over the top.

- Pour over the chocolate custard. Whip the cream until just thick enough to form soft peaks, then place spoonfuls on the custard. Scatter the chocolate flake pieces over the top.

Chocolate Muffin and Custard Sundae

Chop 2 chocolate muffins into chunks and divide between 4 sundae glasses. Add 2 scoops of vanilla ice cream and a scattering of jelly beans to each. Pour over 475 g (15 oz) ready-made chocolate custard and top with a spoonful of extra-thick cream and a few extra jelly beans.

Baked Chocolate Croissant Pudding

Split 4 ready-made croissants in half, spread with 3 tablespoons chocolate hazelnut spread and sandwich back together again. Cut each croissant into 3 pieces and place in a shallow ovenproof dish. Lightly beat 2 eggs with 300 ml (½ pint) chocolate milkshake and pour over the croissants. Bake in a preheated oven, 180°C (350°F), Gas Mark 4, for 20 minutes until the custard has softly set. Serve warm.

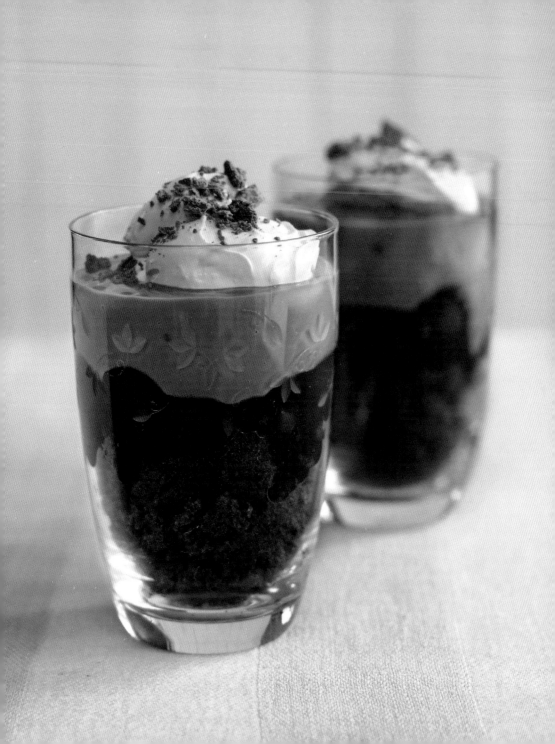

QuickCook
Party time

Recipes listed by cooking time

10

10 Slippery Snake

Serves 8

185 g (6½ oz) can tuna, drained
125 g (4 oz) soft cheese
200 g (7 oz) can sweetcorn, drained
4 bagels, halved
8 cherry tomatoes, halved
1 black grape, halved
1 strip of cucumber skin, cut into a forked tongue

- Mix together the tuna, soft cheese and sweetcorn.

- Cut each bagel half in half again to make 8 semi-circles and arrange them end to end on a board to resemble a curly snake.

- Spread the tuna mixture on the bagels and arrange the cherry tomatoes, cut side down, along the length. Place the grape halves at one end for eyes, and finish with the cucumber forked tongue.

20 Dough Ball Caterpillar

Cook 12 garlic butter dough balls in a preheated oven for 10–15 minutes according to the packet instructions. Arrange in a wiggly line on a bed of mustard and cress. To make ladybirds, place halved plum tomatoes, cut side down, then top with small pieces of black olive stuck on with a little mayonnaise for the spots and eyes.

30 Burger Bugs

Cook 8 burgers under a preheated medium grill according to the packet instructions. Cut 8 burger buns in half and, using scissors, snip the top half of the buns into a zigzag shape to look like teeth. Place the burgers in the buns with lettuce. Arrange 2 halves of a cucumber slice poking out from underneath for feet, then stick 2 cherry tomatoes on cocktail sticks towards the front of the top of the bun to look like 'googly' eyes.

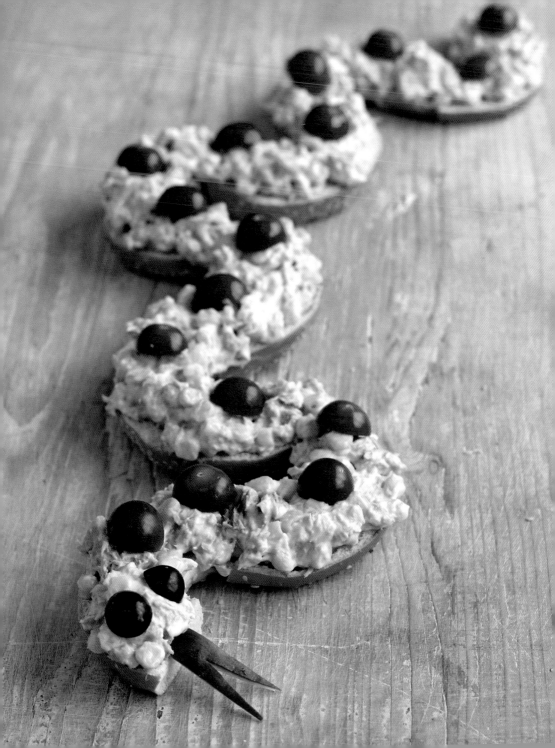

30 Pizza Faces

Makes 4

4 mini pizza bases
300 g (10 oz) ready-made pizza
    sauce
8 thin slices of salami or
    pepperoni
75 g (3 oz) mozzarella cheese,
    grated
4 pitted black olives, halved
2 cherry tomatoes, halved
4 small strips of green pepper
8 strips of red pepper

- Place the pizza bases on a baking sheet and spread the pizza topping over each one, leaving a small border around the edge.

- Place 2 slices of salami or pepperoni on each pizza for eyes, sprinkle with a little mozzarella and place a black olive half in the centre of each one. Add half a cherry tomato for the nose and a strip of green pepper for the mouth.

- Place the red pepper slices at the top for ears, then sprinkle with the remaining mozzarella for hair.

- Bake in a preheated oven, 200°C (400°F), Gas Mark 6, for 10–15 minutes until golden. Serve warm.

1 **Pizza Muffin Faces** Cut 4 English muffins in half and toast both sides. Spread each cut side with a generous teaspoonful of pizza topping sauce, then sprinkle over some grated mozzarella cheese. Grill until golden and arrange cucumber slices, cherry tomatoes and salad leaves to look like faces and hair.

2 **Funny Face Margarita Pizzas** Place a scattering of drained canned sweetcorn to look like hair on 4 ready-made margarita pizzas. Arrange pitted olives for eyes, cherry tomato halves for noses and a strip of salami for a mouth. Place on baking sheets and bake in a preheated oven, 200°C (400°F), Gas Mark 6, for 10 minutes or according to the packet instructions.

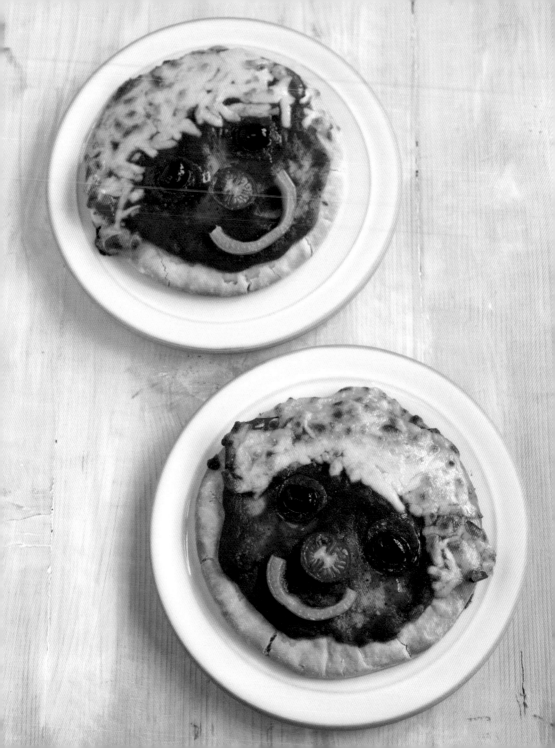

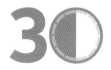

Chocolate and Cranberry Crunch Squares

Makes 9

125 g (4 oz) butter
50 g (2 oz) caster sugar
1 tablespoon golden syrup
4 teaspoons cocoa powder
250 g (8 oz) digestive biscuits, crushed
50 g (2 oz) dried cranberries

For the topping

125 g (4 oz) milk chocolate, broken into pieces
15 g (½ oz) butter
coloured sweets, such as Smarties, to decorate

- Line a shallow 18 cm (7 inch) square tin with clingfilm.

- Melt the butter, sugar, golden syrup and cocoa powder in a saucepan, stirring until smooth. Remove from the heat and stir in the crushed biscuits and cranberries.

- Spoon the mixture into the prepared tin. Press the mixture down firmly and evenly with the back of a spoon. Place in the freezer for 5 minutes to chill.

- To make the topping, heat the chocolate and butter in a heatproof bowl over a saucepan of simmering water, making sure the base of the bowl doesn't touch the water, until melted and smooth.

- Pour the chocolate topping over the biscuit base and spread evenly. Decorate with coloured sweets then return to the freezer for 10 minutes to set. Cut into squares to serve.

10 Rainbow Biscuits Spread digestive biscuits with chocolate hazelnut spread from a jar and sprinkle over cake-decorating confetti dots or mini coloured sweets, such as Smarties.

20 Chocolate and Cranberry Krispie Cakes Heat 250 g (8 oz) plain dark chocolate, broken into pieces with 4 tablespoons golden syrup and 50 g (2 oz) butter in a large heatproof bowl over a saucepan of simmering water, stirring occasionally, until melted and smooth. Stir in 75 g (3 oz) Rice Krispies, or similar cereal, 25 g (1 oz) dried cranberries and 40 g (1½ oz) strawberry fruit flakes. Spoon into paper cake cases and place in the freezer for 5 minutes to set.

KID-PART-SUB

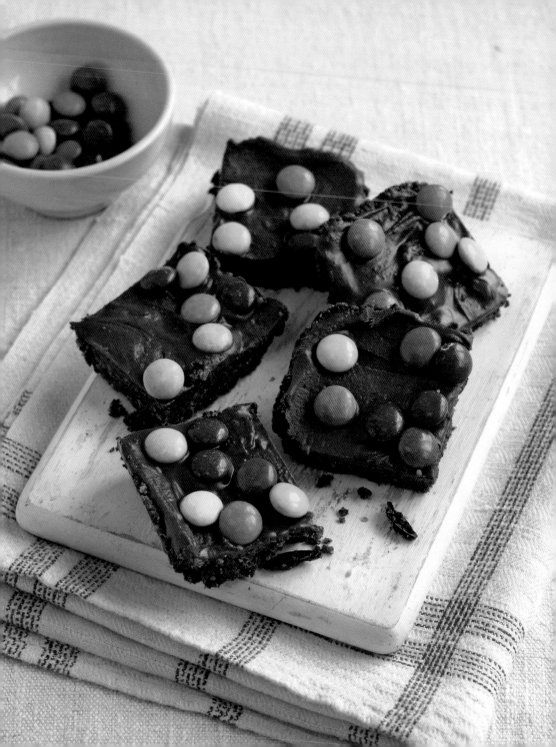

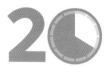

Pirate and Princess Cakes

Makes 12

12 ready-made plain fairy cakes
400 g (13 oz) ready-made
  buttercream icing

For the pirates

50 g (2 oz) red ready-to-roll
  fondant icing
tubes of white and black writing
  icing

For the princesses

mixture of coloured sweets, such
  as dolly mixtures, mini
  marshmallows and cake
  decoration sprinkles
silver ball cake decorations
edible glitter dust (optional)

- For the pirate cakes, spread 6 cakes with buttercream icing and level the surface. Roll out the red icing, cut 6 semi-circles to fit the top third of each cake and place on the cakes to make the scarf hats. Roll any trimmings into little sausages and twists and stick on one side of the hats as knots. Squeeze little dots over the hats, or crossbone shapes, with the white writing icing. Use the black writing icing to make a dot for one eye, an eye patch for the other, a dot for the nose and a large semi-circle for the mouth.

- For the Princess cakes, swirl a generous spoonful of buttercream icing on the top of the 6 remaining cakes. Pile the sweets on top with a few silver balls, then sprinkle with edible glitter dust, if using.

Buried Treasure Cakes

Spread 12 ready-made plain fairy cakes with 400 g (13 oz) ready-made buttercream icing. Put 75 g (3 oz) boiled fruit sweets in a plastic food bag and crush them with a rolling pin. Stick them into the icing with a few silver ball cake decorations.

Treasure Island and Fairytale Castle

Cakes Divide 175 g (6 oz) white ready-to-roll icing in half and knead pink food colouring into one half and green into the other. Roll out the icings and cut 6 circles from each, large enough to cover the tops of 12 ready-made plain fairy cakes. Mix 2 tablespoons icing sugar with a little water to make a smooth icing, spread a little over the top of each cake and stick the rolled-out icing circles on the top. For the fairytale castles, arrange mini marshmallows in a square on the top of each cake, securing with a dot of pink icing. Stick a flag (pink paper stuck on a cocktail stick) in the centre. For the treasure island cakes, sprinkle crushed digestive biscuits around the edge of the green icing for sand. Make palm trees from chocolate finger biscuits and leftover green icing, rolled and snipped for the leaves. Push down into the centre of each cake.

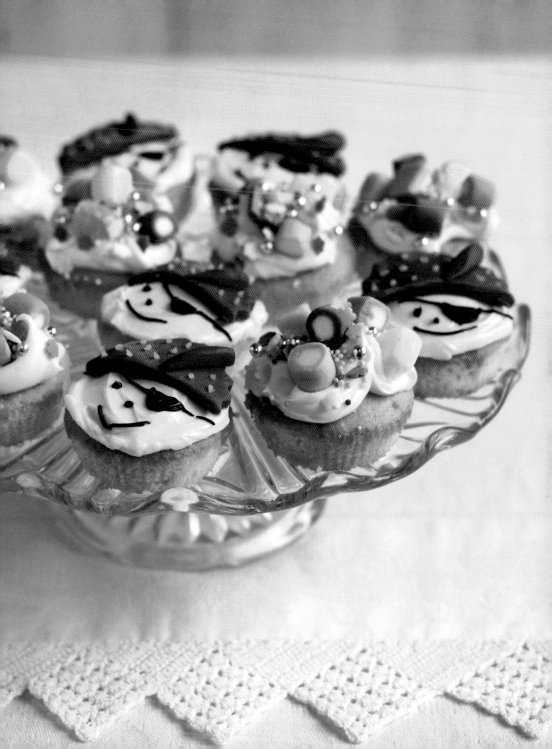

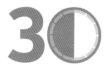

Gingerbread People Beach Party

Makes 6

50 g (2 oz) pink ready-to-roll icing

50 g (2 oz) blue ready-to-roll icing

6 ready-made plain gingerbread men

writing icing tubes in red, black and yellow

125 g (4 oz) demerara sugar

paper cocktail umbrellas

- Roll out the pink and blue icings and cut out bikini shapes for 3 of the gingerbread people and shorts for the other 3. Stick in place with a little of the writing icing. Pipe on faces and hair with the writing icing tubes.

- With the ready-to-roll icing trimmings, re-roll and cut out beach towels, flip flops, beach balls, books, etc.

- Spread the demerara sugar out on a board to make the sand, then arrange the gingerbread people with their towels and accessories and the cocktail umbrellas to make a beach party.

 1 Bow Ties and Hearts Gingerbread Men Roll out 50 g (2 oz) red ready-to-roll icing and cut out 3 hearts large enough to cover the body of 3 ready-made gingerbread men, and 3 large bow ties. Stick on to 6 gingerbread men using a tube of white writing icing and decorate with silver ball cake decorations. Pipe faces with the tube of icing.

 2 Chocolate-Dipped Gingerbread Men Heat 125 g (4 oz) milk chocolate in a heatproof bowl over a saucepan of simmering water, making sure the base of the bowl doesn't touch the water, until melted and smooth. Dip the top of the heads and the toes of 6 ready-made gingerbread men into the chocolate and place on a baking sheet lined with baking paper. Place in the refrigerator for 5 minutes to set. Using a tube of white writing icing, pipe dots for eyes and a nose and a smiling mouth. Stick coloured sweets down the centre for buttons.

KID-PART-FOP

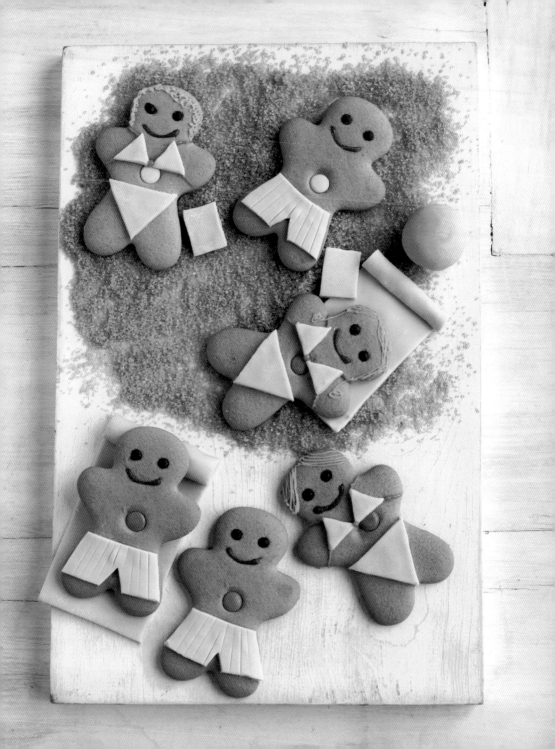

🕙 Mocktails

Each mocktail serves 2

Fizzy Fish
6 fizzy fish sweets
150 ml (¼ pint) mango juice
chilled lemonade

Paradise Cooler
300 ml (½ pint) pineapple juice
2 scoops of vanilla ice cream

Beach Babes
150 ml (¼ pint) orange juice
150 ml (¼ pint) cranberry juice
  drink
sparkling mineral water
2 orange slices, to decorate
2 strawberries, to decorate

- For the Fizzy Fish, place the sweets in the bottom of 2 tumblers. Add the mango juice and top up with lemonade. Serve with cocktail sticks to see who can 'fish' out the sweets first.

- For the Paradise Cooler, pour the pineapple juice into 2 glasses and top each with a scoop of ice cream. Decorate with cocktail umbrellas and long spoons to eat the ice cream.

- For the Beach Babes, divide the juices between 2 glasses, top up with sparkling water and decorate the rim of the each glass with an orange slice and a strawberry.

2🕙 Swampy Punch
Put 10 grapes in the freezer for 15 minutes to get really cold. In a bowl or jug, mix together 4 tablespoons blackcurrant squash and 600 ml (1 pint) cola. Add 4 scoops of chocolate ice cream and add some spider sweets and jelly worms. Add the semi-frozen grapes just before serving. Pour into glasses and decorate with extra jelly worms.

3🕙 Mixed Berry and Apple Smoothies
with Vegetable Crisps Using a vegetable peeler, cut 1 parsnip, 1 carrot and 1 sweet potato into thin ribbons. Dry on kitchen paper, then place in a bowl with 2 tablespoons olive oil. Season with salt and pepper and mix well to coat. Spread the slices out over a large baking sheet and cook in a preheated oven, 220°C (425°F), Gas Mark 7, for

about 5 minutes until golden and crisp. To make the smoothie, blend 250 g (8 oz) hulled strawberries, 175 g (6 oz) frozen raspberries and 3 peeled, cored and quartered dessert apples in a food processor until smooth. Add 300 ml (½ pint) orange juice and blend again. Pour into glasses and place a strawberry on the rim of each glass. Serve with the vegetable crisps.

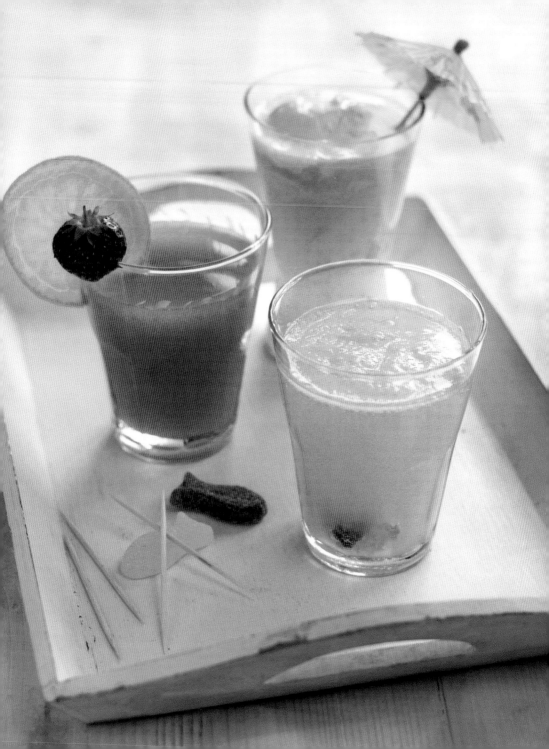

1 Magic Wands

Makes 10

75 g (3 oz) white chocolate,
  broken into pieces
10 breadsticks
multicoloured cake decoration
  sprinkles

- Put a baking sheet lined with baking paper into the freezer to chill.

- Heat the chocolate in a heatproof bowl over a saucepan of simmering water, making sure the base of the bowl doesn't touch the water, until melted and smooth. Pour into a mug (this gives more depth of chocolate for dipping).

- Dip one end of each breadstick into the chocolate and shake off any excess. Roll in the sprinkles and place on the cold baking sheet. Return to the freezer for a few minutes to set.

2 Glitter Stars

Unroll 325 g (11 oz) ready-rolled sweet dessert pastry and cut out star shapes using a 7 cm (3 inch) cutter. Place on a baking sheet and bake in a preheated oven, 190°C (375°F), Gas Mark 5, for 10 minutes until golden and crisp. Mix 125 g (4 oz) icing sugar with about 2 teaspoons water to make a smooth icing. Drizzle over the biscuits and sprinkle with multicoloured cake decoration sprinkles and a dusting of edible glitter.

3 Yum Yum Twists

Unroll a 250 g (8 oz) canned croissant dough. Cut the dough into 12 strips widthways. Twist 2 strips together, securing the ends with a dab of water, then place on a baking sheet. Repeat to make 6 twists. Brush with a little milk and bake in a preheated oven, 200°C (400°F), Gas Mark 6, for about 10 minutes until golden. Mix 125 g (4 oz) icing sugar with about 1 tablespoon water to make a smooth runny icing. Drizzle over the yum yums and sprinkle over multicoloured cake decoration sprinkles.

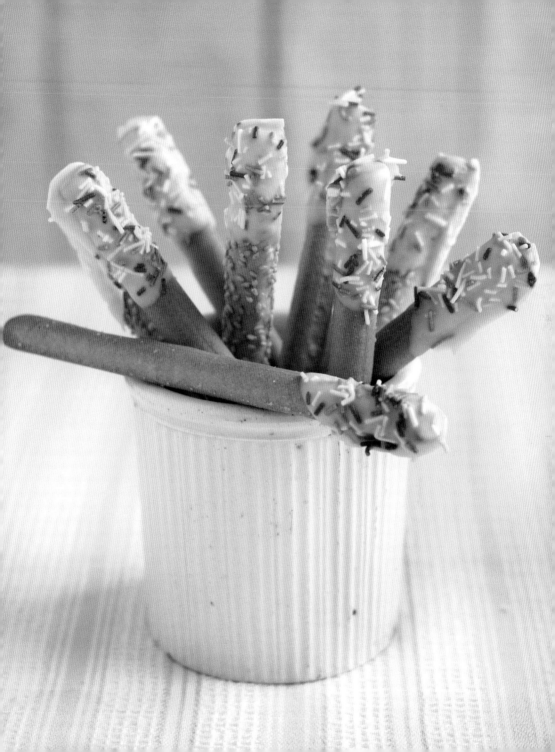

20 Number Biscuits

Makes about 10

325 g (11 oz) ready-rolled sweet
dessert pastry
4 tablespoons strawberry jam
icing sugar, for dusting

- Unroll the pastry and cut out numbers using large biscuit cutters, cutting each number twice.

- Place on baking sheets and bake in a preheated oven, 190°C (375°F), Gas Mark 5, for 10 minutes until golden and crisp.

- Place the numbers together in pairs. Spread one with a layer of jam and top with the other. Dust with icing sugar and arrange together significant numbers to make dates such as birthdays or ages.

---

10 Message Biscuits

Arrange coloured sweets on ready-made chocolate digestive biscuits to form a letter on each biscuit. Stick in place with a dab of icing from a tube of writing icing. Arrange the biscuits to spell out your chosen name or message.

30 Lollipop Biscuits

Unroll 325 g (11 oz) ready-rolled sweet dessert pastry and cut out 12 rounds using a 7 cm (3 inch) cutter. Place on 2 baking sheets and carefully push a wooden lolly stick into the side of each round to reach the centre. Bake in a preheated oven, 190°C (375°F), Gas Mark 5, for 10 minutes until golden. While the biscuits are cooking, roll out 125 g (4 oz) pink or blue ready-to-roll icing and cut out numbers or letters using biscuit cutters. Stick the numbers or letters on to the biscuits with a dab of icing from a tube of writing icing and decorate with coloured sweets.

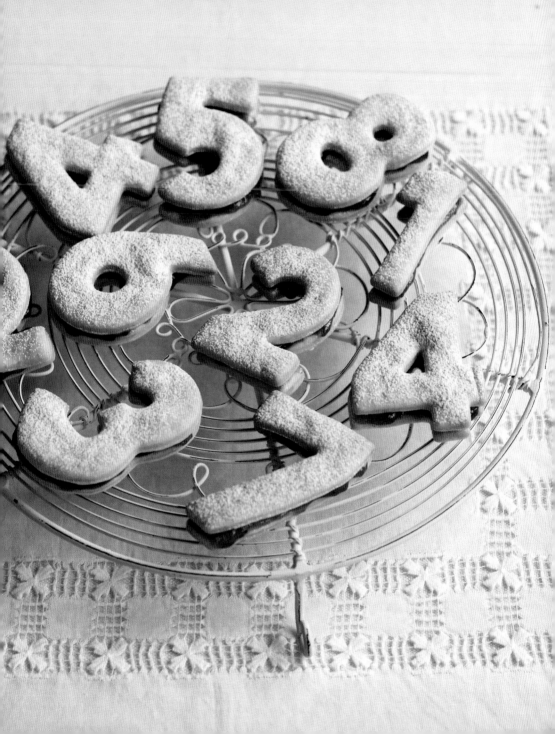

1⃝ Cheesy Garlic Bread

Serves 8

1 French stick

125 g (4 oz) ready-made garlic and herb butter

200 g (7 oz) mozzarella cheese, grated

- Cut the French stick in half lengthways. Spread the garlic and herb butter generously over both halves and place on a baking sheet (cut the bread in half if it is too long for the oven).

- Sprinkle over the mozzarella and bake in a preheated oven, 220°C (425°F), Gas Mark 7, for 5 minutes until the cheese has melted. Cut into pieces to serve.

 2 Garlic and Herb Flatbread with Cheese Dip Melt 50 g (2 oz) butter in a saucepan or in the microwave with 1 crushed garlic clove. Remove from the heat and stir in 1 tablespoon chopped parsley. Brush the mixture over a ready-made pizza base and bake in a preheated oven, 200°C (400°F), Gas Mark 6, for 10 minutes until crisp and golden. Cut into wedges and serve with a dip made from 125 g (4 oz) garlic and herb soft cheese beaten with 2 tablespoons milk.

 3 Cheesy Garlic Ciabatta Beat 125 g (4 oz) softened butter with 2 crushed garlic cloves and 2 tablespoons chopped parsley. Season with salt and pepper. Cut a ciabatta loaf into 1 cm (½ inch) slices, but don't cut all the way through. Spread the butter on both sides of each slice. Cut 150 g (5 oz) mozzarella cheese into slices and insert a piece of cheese between each slice of bread. Wrap the loaf in foil and cook in a preheated oven, 200°C (400°F), Gas Mark 6, for 15 minutes until hot and crispy and the cheese has melted. Unwrap, cut through the slices and serve warm while the cheese is still gooey.

KID-PART-DOO

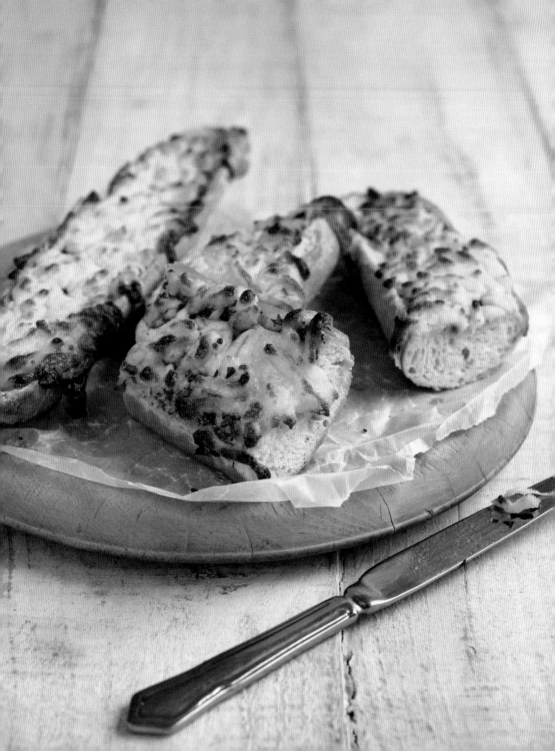

3⦿ Whirly Sausage Rolls

Makes 12

200 g (7 oz) ready-rolled puff
   pastry
16 chipolata sausages
beaten egg, to glaze
1 tablespoon sesame seeds
ketchup, to serve

- Unroll the pastry and cut into 12 x 1.5 cm (¾ inch) strips widthways.

- Wind a strip of pastry around each sausage and place on a baking sheet. Brush with beaten egg and sprinkle over a few sesame seeds.

- Bake in a preheated oven, 200°C (400°F), Gas Mark 6, for 20 minutes until the pastry is well risen and golden and the sausages are cooked. Serve warm with ketchup for dipping.

1⦿ Barbecue Sausage Wraps

Cook 12 chipolatas under a preheated grill for 5 minutes, turning occasionally, until almost cooked. Brush with 2 tablespoons barbecue sauce and cook for a further 2–3 minutes until sticky and beginning to char. Warm 6 flour tortillas in the microwave according to the packet instructions. Place 2 sausages on each, together with crisp Little Gem lettuce leaves and a sprinkling of sweetcorn. Roll up the wraps to enclose the filling and serve in paper napkins.

2⦿ Cheese and Bacon Hot Dogs

Cook 6 sausages under a preheated grill for 10 minutes, turning occasionally, until cooked through. Using tongs to hold them, carefully cut a slit along the length of each sausage. Cut 3 cheese slices each into 4 strips and place 2 strips in the slit in each sausage. Wrap a bacon rasher around each sausage and grill for 5 minutes until the bacon is cooked. Serve in hot dog rolls with ketchup.

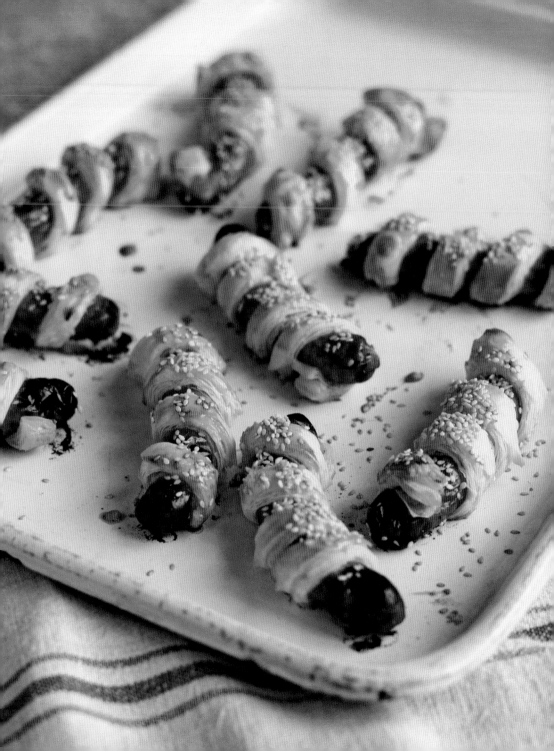

10 Rocky Road Popcorn

Serves 4

2 tablespoons sunflower oil
75 g (3 oz) popping corn
75 g (3 oz) butter
4 tablespoons instant hot
  chocolate powder
75 g (3 oz) mini marshmallows

- Put the oil and popping corn into a large saucepan. Cover with a tight-fitting lid and place the pan over a medium heat. Leave for 2–3 minutes until you hear the first pop. Shake the pan firmly, keeping the lid in place and the pan on the heat.

- When the popping stops, remove from the heat and tip the popcorn into a bowl. Add the butter to the pan with the chocolate powder and heat to melt. Pour over the popcorn and stir well.

- Add the marshmallows and serve in paper cones or cups.

 Popcorn Necklaces
Cook 300 g (10 oz) microwave butter popcorn according to the packet instructions. Tip into a bowl. Thread the popcorn, together with seedless grapes and mini marshmallows, on to lengths of thread using a blunt tapestry needle. Tie the ends of the thread in a knot to secure.

 Malteser Popcorn Balls
Heat 2 tablespoons vegetable oil in a large saucepan with 75 g (3 oz) popping corn. Cover with a tight-fitting lid and cook, shaking the pan occasionally, until the popping stops. Tip the popcorn into a bowl. Melt 125 g (4 oz) butter in the hot pan with 150 g (5 oz) golden caster sugar and 1 tablespoon golden syrup. Bring to the boil and simmer for about 5 minutes until golden. Pour over the popcorn, mix well and stir in 75 g (3 oz) roughly chopped Maltesers. Spoon into balls and place on a baking sheet lined with baking paper. Chill in the freezer for 10 minutes.

KID-PART-NAY

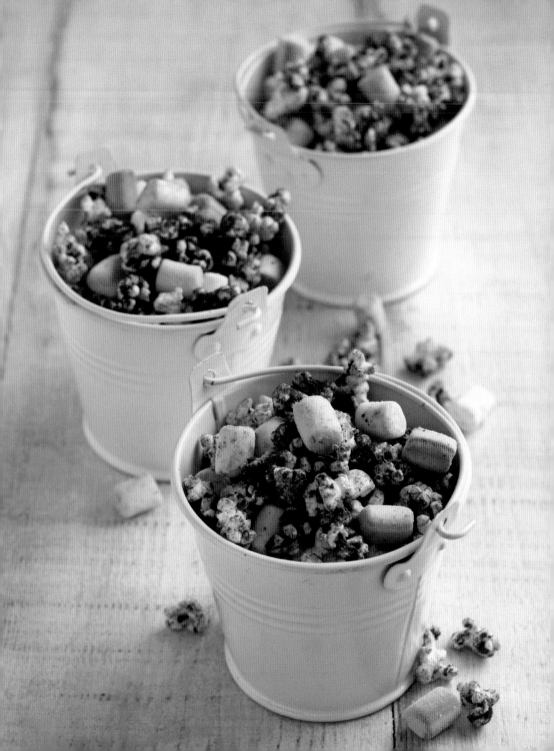

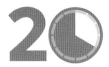

Flower Garden Sandwiches

Serves 8

2 teaspoons Marmite or other
  yeast extract
200 g (7 oz) soft cheese
8 slices of white bread
8 slices of brown bread
2 cherry tomatoes, halved
2 green grapes, halved
1 punnet mustard and cress
1 large carrot, peeled and sliced

- Mix together the Marmite and soft cheese in a bowl, then spread over the white bread. Cover with the brown bread and press together firmly. Using a medium-sized cutter, cut out as many flower shapes as you can.

- Cut a small circle out of the centre of each sandwich using an apple corer and stick either a cherry tomato half or grape half in the middle.

- Arrange on a plate or board on a bed of mustard and cress. Cut small flower shapes from the carrot slices using a small cutter and scatter over the 'grass'.

Ham Sticks

Thinly spread a little marmite or other yeast extract down one side of 12 breadsticks. Cut 6 slices of wafer-thin ham into strips and wrap around the breadsticks pressing on to the marmite to help it stick. Serve with a selection of raw vegetables such as carrots, mangetout and celery.

Party Whirls

Unroll 325 g (11 oz) ready-rolled puff pastry and spread with marmite or other yeast extract. Sprinkle over 125 g (4 oz) grated Cheddar cheese and loosely roll up, starting with one long side. Cut into slices, place on 2 baking sheets lined with baking paper and bake in a preheated oven, 200°C (400°F), Gas Mark 6, for 15 minutes until golden.

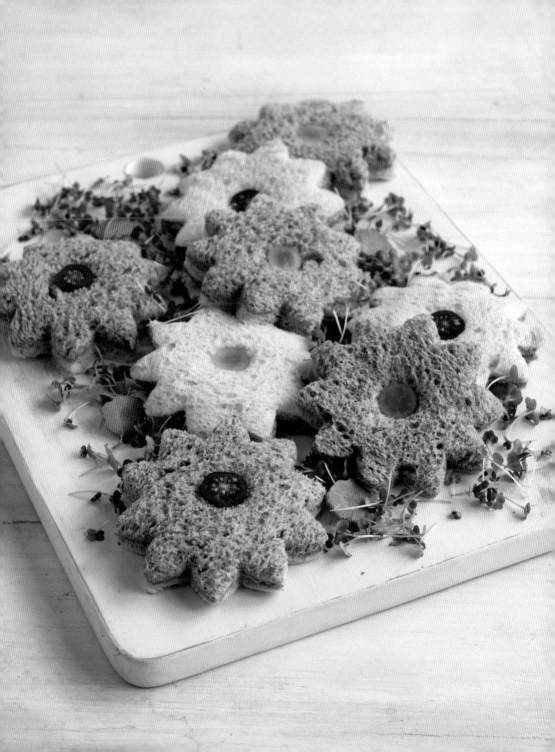

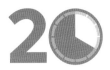

BLT Club Sandwiches

Makes 8

4 back bacon rashers
6 slices of wholemeal bread
1 carrot, peeled and grated
125 g (4 oz) soft cheese
2 tomatoes, sliced
6 Little Gem lettuce leaves
cherry tomatoes and cucumber
   sticks, to serve

- Cook the bacon under a preheated hot grill for about 5 minutes, turning once, until crisp.

- Toast the bread slices on both sides.

- Mix together the carrot and soft cheese and spread over 2 slices of the toast. Arrange the tomato slices on top.

- Cover with another slice of toast, and top with the lettuce and bacon. Place the remaining slices of toast on top.

- Press the sandwich stacks down firmly and cut each into 4 triangles. Stick a cocktail stick flag through each sandwich to hold it all together. Serve with halved cherry tomatoes and cucumber sticks.

Sandwich Kebabs

Cut one-quarter of a French stick into chunks, making sure each piece has some crust on it. Thread on to wooden skewers with cherry tomatoes, cubes of cheese, chunks of cucumber and ready-cooked cocktail sausages.

Surprise Rolls

Cut a slice off the top of 6 round bread rolls and keep the slices for lids. Pull out most of the soft bread from the inside of each roll (this can be saved for making breadcrumbs and frozen), leaving a hollow roll. Lightly brush the inside of the rolls with melted butter, then layer up the filling. Between the rolls, divide 4 chopped grilled bacon rashers, 2 sliced tomatoes, 4 small lettuce leaves and 125 g (4 oz) soft cheese mixed with 1 grated carrot. Press the filling down firmly and replace the lids.

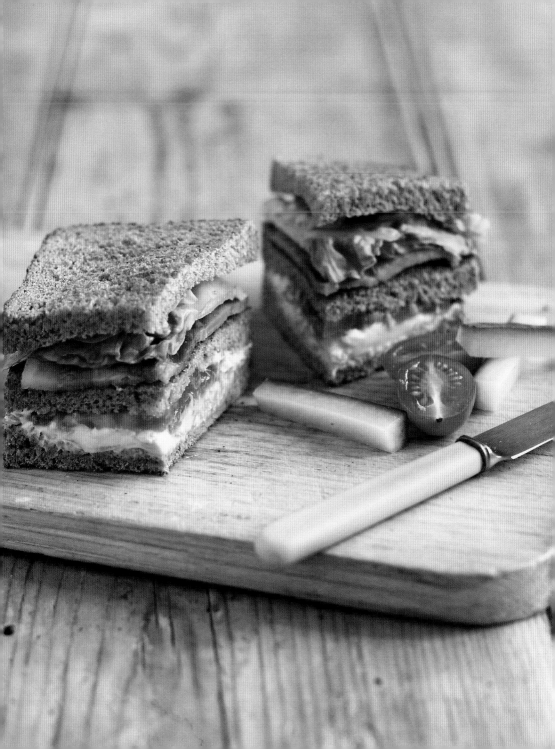

30 Mini Fish and Chip Cones

Serves 6

2 baking potatoes, about 175 g
   (6 oz) each, scrubbed
4 tablespoons sunflower oil
400 g (13 oz) skinless chunky
   white fish fillets, cut into
   bite-sized pieces
2 tablespoons plain flour
1 egg, beaten
125 g (4 oz) ready-made or dried
   natural breadcrumbs
salt and pepper

- Cut the potatoes into thin sticks, coat in 2 tablespoons of the oil and spread out over a baking sheet. Bake in a preheated oven, 220°C (425°F), Gas Mark 7, for 20 minutes, turning occasionally, until golden and cooked through. Season with salt and pepper.

- Meanwhile, place the flour on one plate, the beaten egg on another and the breadcrumbs on a third. Dip the fish pieces in the flour, then the egg and finally the breadcrumbs, pressing firmly to coat.

- Heat the remaining oil in a frying pan and cook the fish for 5 minutes, turning occasionally, until golden, crisp and cooked through.

- Divide the chips between paper cones made from greaseproof paper and top with the pieces of fish.

10 Fish Finger Pittas

Cook 8 fish fingers under a preheated medium grill for 5–8 minutes, turning occasionally, until golden and cooked through. Cut in half and use to fill warmed mini pitta breads with some lettuce and a spoonful of soured cream and chive dip on each.

20 Fish and Chip Butties

Place 8 fish fingers and 175 g (6 oz) thin-cut oven chips on a baking sheet and cook in a preheated oven, 220°C (425°F), Gas Mark 7, for 15 minutes, turning once, until golden and cooked. Split 4 soft white submarine rolls and fill with the fish fingers, chips, a few lettuce leaves and cucumber slices and a squirt of ketchup.

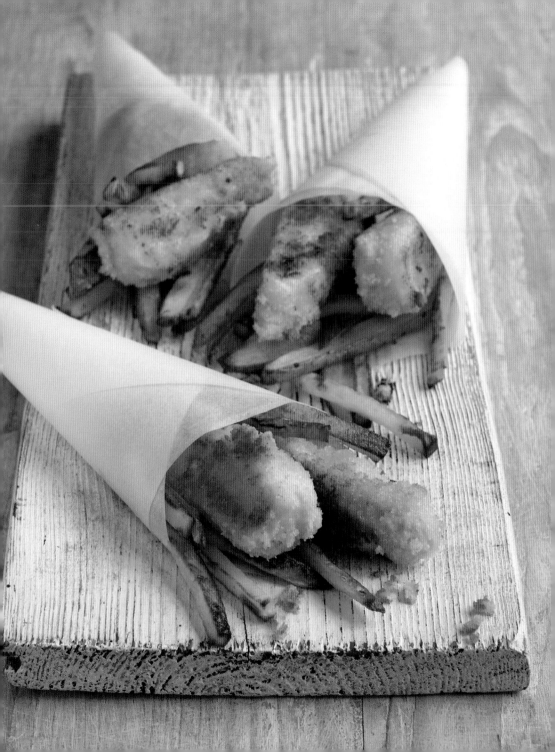

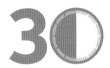

Dolly Mixture Tray Bake

Makes 12

175 g (6 oz) sunflower spread
175 g (6 oz) caster sugar
3 eggs, beaten
175 g (6 oz) self-raising flour
125 g (6 oz) icing sugar
1½ tablespoons lemon juice
dolly mixture sweets, to decorate

- Line a shallow 18 x 28 cm (7 x 11 inch) baking tin with baking paper.

- Beat together the sunflower spread, caster sugar, eggs and flour until soft and creamy. Spoon the mixture into the tin, spread the surface level and bake in a preheated oven, 190°C (375°F), Gas Mark 5, for 20 minutes until golden and just firm to the touch.

- Mix together the icing sugar and lemon juice to make a smooth, runny icing, then drizzle over the cake with a teaspoon.

- Cut into 12 squares or fingers and pile a few dolly mixtures on top of each.

 Dolly Mixture Squares

Cut a Madeira loaf cake into 2.5 cm (1 inch) cubes. Melt 3 tablespoons lemon curd with 1 tablespoon water in a pan and stir until smooth. Brush the lemon curd over the cubes, then roll in desiccated coconut. Top with a few dolly mixtures.

 Dolly Mixture 'Pizza'

Unroll 325 g (11 oz) ready-rolled sweet dessert pastry and cut out the largest circle you can, using a plate as a guide. Place on a baking sheet and bake in a preheated oven, 200°C (400°F), Gas Mark 6, for 10 minutes until golden. Spread with 3 tablespoons lemon curd and scatter fruit and dolly mixtures over the top.

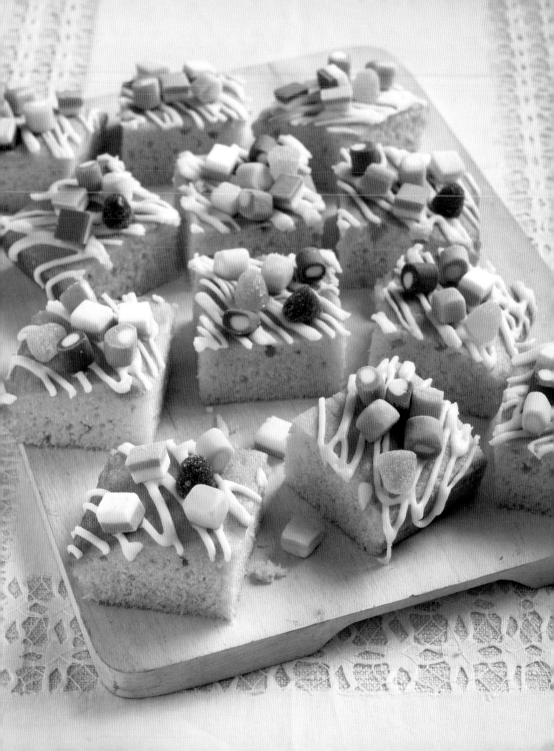

Index

Page references in *italics* indicate photographs

Acknowledgements

Recipes by **Emma Jane Frost**
Executive Editor **Eleanor Maxfield**
Editor **Jo Wilson**
Copy Editor **Alison Copland**
Art Direction **Tracy Killick & Geoff Fennell for Tracy Killick Art Direction and Design**
Original design concept **www.gradedesign.com**
Designer **Geoff Fennell for Tracy Killick Art Direction and Design**
Photographer **William Reavell**
Home Economist **Emma Jane Frost**
Prop Stylist **Liz Hippisley**
Production **Davide Pontiroli**